12-LEAD EKG CONFIDENCE

Second Edition

About the Authors

Jacqueline M. Green, MS, RN, APN-C, CNS, CCRN

Jacqueline Green received her BS in Nursing from Kean University. She attended Rutgers University where she received an MS in Nursing. She is presently a Clinical Nurse Specialist–Cardiac Services at Robert Wood Johnson University Hospital in New Brunswick NJ.

Anthony J. Chiaramida, MD, FACC

Dr. Chiaramida received his BS in Chemistry from Fordham University. He attended the University of Southern California School of Medicine, where he graduated with honors as a member of AOA. He completed his internship and residency at Cornell Cooperating Hospitals (North Shore–Memorial Sloan Kettering). He completed his training in Cardiology at Emory University and is a Fellow of the American College of Physicians and the American College of Cardiology. Since completing his studies in Cardiology at Emory University, he has taught the monthly fourth-year medical student EKG elective to Robert Wood Johnson Medical School students. He makes teaching rounds daily in the CCU and ICU with students, nurses, respiratory therapists, dieticians, interns, and residents.

12-LEAD EKG CONFIDENCE

A Step-by-Step Guide

Second Edition

Jacqueline M. Green, MS, RN, APN-C, CNS, CCRN
Anthony J. Chiaramida, MD, FACC

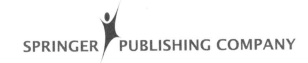
SPRINGER PUBLISHING COMPANY

Springer Publishing Company, LLC
11 West 42nd Street
New York, NY 10036
www.springerpub.com

Acquisitions Editor: Margaret Zuccarini
Production Editor: Barbara A. Chernow
Cover design: Steve Pisano
Composition: Agnew's, Inc.

Ebook ISBN: 978-0-8261-0473-1

09 10 11 12/ 5 4 3 2 1

Library of Congress Cataloging-in-Publication Data
Green, Jacqueline M.
   12-lead EKG confidence : a step-by-step guide / Jacqueline M. Green, Anthony J. Chiaramida. — 2nd ed.
      p. ; cm.
   Includes index.
   ISBN 978-0-8261-0472-4
   1. Electrocardiography.   I. Chiaramida, Anthony J.   II. Title.   III. Title: Twelve-lead EKG confidence.
   [DNLM: 1. Electrocardiography—methods—Programmed Instruction. WG 18.2 G796z 2009]
   RC683.5.E5.G685   2009
   616.1'207547—dc22   2009028242

Printed in the United States of America by Bang Printing.

To my children, Caroline and Conor, with Love always . . .

And to you Phil,
who encouraged me, read every paper I ever wrote, and
who sacrificed the most . . . Thank You

—J.G.

To my mom, who taught me how. And to my dad, who taught me why . . .
and to my children, Jennifer, Joseph, and Matthew,
who teach me anything else that really matters.

—A.C.

CONTENTS

Section VII: The Non-Ischemic Disorders: EKG Changes Related to Drugs, Electrolyte Abnormalities, and Other Diseases

Section VIII: Self-Assessment

In many ways, teaching is like taking students on a train ride. The goal of a teacher is to get the trainload of students from New York to California, without losing anyone along the way. The train ride cannot take forever, but if it travels too quickly, students "fall off" the train, and the excursion is for naught. The train ride also cannot have too many side stops, or too few. The train should arrive at a destination clear to the student and teacher alike. The teacher must have a clear vision and, hopefully, travels a well-worn path to that end. Our goal here is to teach the ability to form an autonomous and clinically useful opinion about any 12 lead EKG. Many books exist. Some are short easy rides that do not get to the destination we envision. Others are laborious tomes that serve for reference only.

We believe this book is unique because it uses a step-by-step method, reinforced by practice EKGs, until by the end, the student is forming a complete autonomous opinion about a selection of 12-lead EKGs. We expect the student to be successful, because we have used this method for 20 years with a variety of students. It is an achievable goal. We have taken students there many times. The opinion the student forms will be based on understanding, which always makes memorization simpler. Other EKG books typically rely on EKG interpretation by pattern memorization and never discuss the basis for these patterns.

The first section of the book discusses basic principles of anatomy and physiology, including a review of the heart's electrical system. It is not an exhaustive introduction and sacrifices density for clarity. The remaining chapters introduce one concept at a time and build on them with each subsequent chapter.

Each chapter is followed by a practice session of 12-lead EKGs. We expect the student to form an opinion on the EKG and then give a clinically meaningful correlation. Upon completion of the book, the reader should be able to confidently work through the entire answer sheet, forming an autonomous useful opinion about a 12-lead EKG.

Each of these includes an analysis by both authors. Another feature of the book is that each EKG opinion refers back directly to the patient, with diagnostic possibilities. Included in our EKG analysis is useful, pertinent, hands-on clinical information relevant to daily practice. The last chapter of the book is a collection of practice EKGs that includes material covered in all the previous chapters. By the end of the book, the reader should have the knowledge and skills to interpret the entire EKG.

All the nurses, doctors, and students who made so many great suggestions for improvement from the original edition.

—A.C. and J.G.

Heart disease has been the leading cause of death in the United States for the last 80 years, responsible for more than 2,500 deaths every day. The 12-lead EKG is a standard test for patients with heart disease and symptoms suggestive of heart disease. Patients who are transported in ambulances, present to emergency rooms (ERs), get admitted to telemetry units, or go to the operating rooms (ORs), invariably have a full 12-lead EKG, as well as constant rhythm monitoring.

The first responders in the field, or in the ER, frequently receive the EKG from the tech. Yet, they have little confidence in their ability to diagnose major problems on the EKG. In hospital critical care units, it is the nurse who sees the rhythm strip or the full 12-lead EKG when the patient first has a change in status.

Major manufacturers of Critical Care/OR/ER/Paramedic monitors now supply the ability to record the full 12-lead EKG in addition to rhythms. This will increase the need for the "first line personnel," typically nurses, to be confident in their ability to interpret a full 12-lead EKG.

Our book addresses such a need. The methodology has been field tested for over 20 years by Dr. Chiaramida, in his fourth-year medical school elective for students at the Robert Wood Johnson Medical School. The elective has been perennially popular; its enrollment includes nearly half the graduating class. Dr. Chiaramida also conducts daily teaching rounds in the critical care units of Raritan Bay Medical Center and has been teaching nurses for over 20 years as well. This background has enabled him to see the needs of the nurse in the unit, as well as the successful techniques that have made him popular as an instructor.

This book supplies a complete approach to the needs of the student nurse, medical student, or practicing nurse. It is a step-by-step approach, with organized sections leading to self-assessment tests with real world, full 12-lead EKGs. The book is totally goal oriented. Jacqueline Green has a 20-year history in cardiac education and brings dramatic clarity and focus to the practical clinical usefulness of the skills taught in this book. She brings all the skill, expertise, knowledge, understanding, and clinical relevance that her position as APN-C at the Robert Wood Johnson University Hospital Critical Care Unit demands on a daily basis. We believe it is a unique and very successful collaboration.

1) Check the P wave direction to make sure the EKG was taken correctly.
2) Measure the HR and interpret it clinically. It is always relevant.
3) Measure the QRS. Diagnose BBB if it is ≥0.12 seconds. Diagnose right or left bundle by looking only at the end of the QRS. Do not diagnose LVH, RVH, ischemia, or infarction with LBBB.
4) Visualize the overall QRS direction. Diagnose hemiblock if the QRS points superiorly (LAHB) or rightward (LPHB).
5) Measure the QT interval, and check the corrected QT (QTc) against a chart. This can be a clue to dangerous drug or electrolyte toxicity.
6) The First Rule of the T Wave: On a single EKG, neither T wave inversion nor ST depression proves either timing or reversibility.
7) The Second Rule of the T wave: When both ST depression and T wave inversion are present, ST depression takes precedence. It is more specific and carries a worse prognosis.
8) The Third Rule of the T wave: When ST elevation is present in two contiguous leads it takes precedence over ST depression and T wave inversion. Therapeutic intervention should be instituted ASAP to open the artery.
9) Q waves evolve from undertreated ST elevation pathophysiology. Interpret associated T or ST segment abnormalities according to the Three Rules of the T waves.
10) LVH can cause ST changes and PRWP due to the hypertrophy process or due to consequent coronary disease.
11) Anterior ST depression may be due to LV disease in the septum or posterior wall, or to RV strain due to acute pulmonary embolism.
12) Specific patterns of hyperkalemia, pericarditis, and pulmonary embolism should be looked for on every EKG.

Overview of Heart Function and the EKG

I

Anatomy Review
of the Human Heart

Anatomy of the Heart: Overview

The human heart is a hollow four-chambered muscle that is responsible for pumping blood throughout the body. The heart lies in the mediastinum in the thorax, pointing slightly toward the left of the midline.

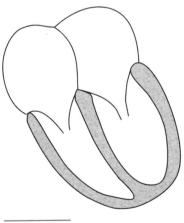

FIGURE 1.1

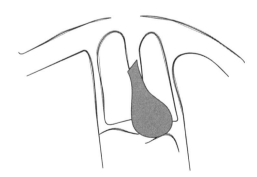

FIGURE 1.2

Self-Study Objectives

◼ **Define and identify the following:**

Pericardium

Myocardium

Endocardium

Epicardium

Circulation

Origin and path of the right coronary artery

Origin and path of the left coronary artery

Branches of the left coronary artery

Blood supply to the right ventricle

Blood supply to the AV node

Blood supply to the septum, anterior wall, lateral walls, posterior wall, and inferior wall of the heart

The Pericardium

The heart consists of four main layers: the pericardium, epicardium, myocardium, and endocardium. The pericardium is a loose fitting fibroserous sac that covers the heart. Separating the epicardium, the outermost layer of the heart muscle from the pericardium, is a space called the pericardial space. The space is filled with fluid which acts as a lubricating agent protecting the heart from injuries caused by friction while it is beating.

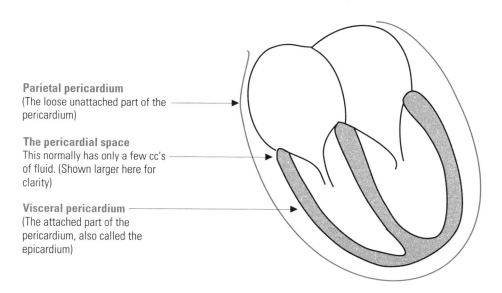

Parietal pericardium
(The loose unattached part of the pericardium)

The pericardial space
This normally has only a few cc's of fluid. (Shown larger here for clarity)

Visceral pericardium
(The attached part of the pericardium, also called the epicardium)

FIGURE 1.3

Layers of the Heart

The epicardium is the outermost layer of the heart muscle. It also is known as the visceral pericardium. The middle layer of the heart is called the myocardium. The myocardium is the thick muscular layer of the heart and is responsible for the heart's ability to contract. The innermost layer of the heart is the endocardium. This layer lines the valves and chambers of the heart.

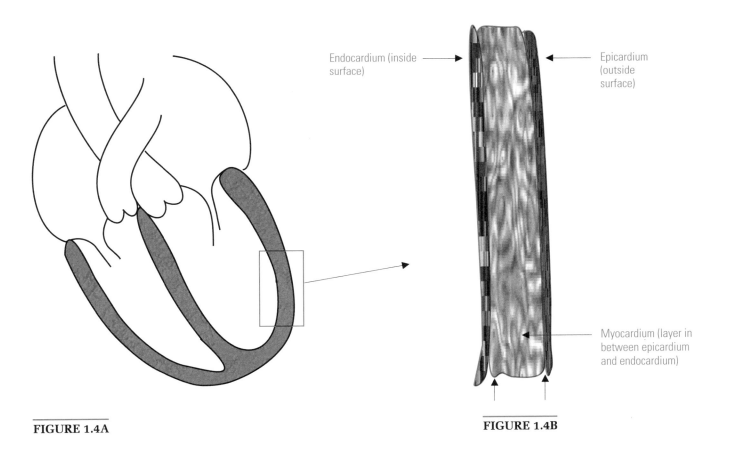

Endocardium (inside surface)

Epicardium (outside surface)

Myocardium (layer in between epicardium and endocardium)

FIGURE 1.4A

FIGURE 1.4B

Heart Chambers

The heart is divided into two sides; the right side and the left side. The right side of the heart contains the right atrium and right ventricle. The left side of the heart contains the left atrium and left ventricle. The right and left sides of the heart are anatomically separated by the atrial septum and the ventricular septum. The two sides of the heart could be considered two separate pumps and essentially work independently of each other.

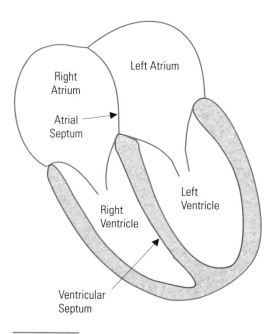

FIGURE 1.5

The Circulation

The right atrium receives deoxygenated blood from the body via the superior and inferior venae cavae. During diastole, the blood is pushed from the right atrium into the right ventricle. The blood is then forced out of the right ventricle into the pulmonary circulation where it picks up oxygen. The oxygen-rich blood is transported into the left atrium via the pulmonary veins. During ventricular diastole, the blood is forced into the left ventricle. The left ventricle pumps the oxygen-rich blood throughout the body.

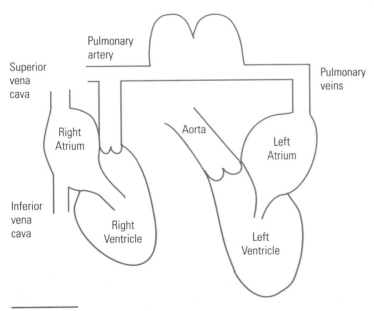

FIGURE 1.6

The Heart Valves

The heart has four valves that act as tiny doors that keep the blood moving in one direction. The closure of the valves prevents the backward flow of blood. The right atrium and right ventricle are separated by the tricuspid valve and the left atrium and left ventricle are separated by the mitral valve. These valves are known as cuspid valves. The aortic valve lies between the left ventricle and the aorta, and the pulmonic valve separates the right ventricle from the pulmonary artery. The aortic and pulmonic valves are called semilunar valves because of their distinct half-moon appearance.

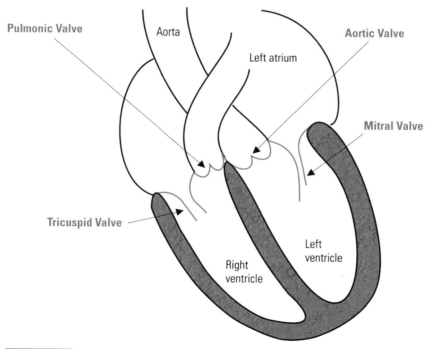

FIGURE 1.7

The Coronary Circulation

The heart muscle receives oxygen-rich blood via two main vessels: the right coronary artery (RCA) and the left coronary artery (LCA). Both arteries arise from the aortic root. As they travel down the length of the heart, each divides into several branches, as shown below.

The right coronary artery (RCA) originates at the aortic root, travels around the front of the right ventricle. It loops around to the back of the right ventricle, and then, when it meets the back of the septum, it turns to the apex.

The left coronary artery (LCA) begins at the aortic root, and splits into the LAD (left anterior descending) and CFX (circumflex) branches. The LAD goes down the front of the septum. The circumflex goes left, around to the back of the left ventricle.

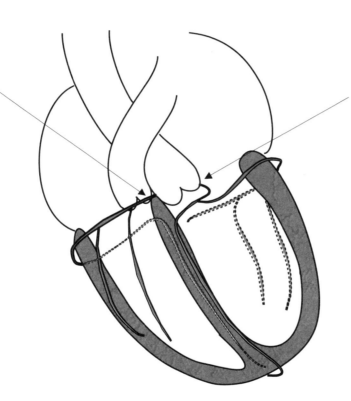

FIGURE 1.8

The Right Coronary Artery

The right coronary artery travels along the coronary sulcus, which is the groove between the atria and the ventricles, and continues down the posterior aspect of the ventricular septum. It supplies blood to the right ventricle, the atrioventricular (AV) node, part of the septum, as well as to the posterior and inferior walls of the left ventricle.

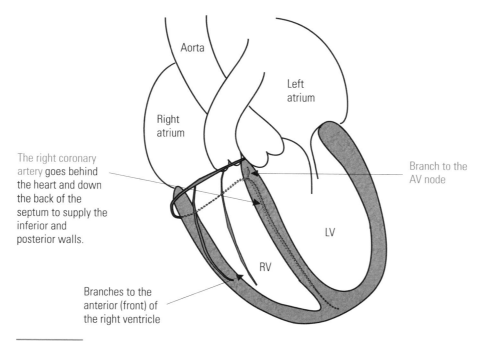

The right coronary artery goes behind the heart and down the back of the septum to supply the inferior and posterior walls.

Branch to the AV node

Branches to the anterior (front) of the right ventricle

Aorta

Left atrium

Right atrium

LV

RV

FIGURE 1.9

The Left Coronary Artery

The left coronary artery consists of two branches, the left anterior descending branch (LAD) and the circumflex branch (CFX).

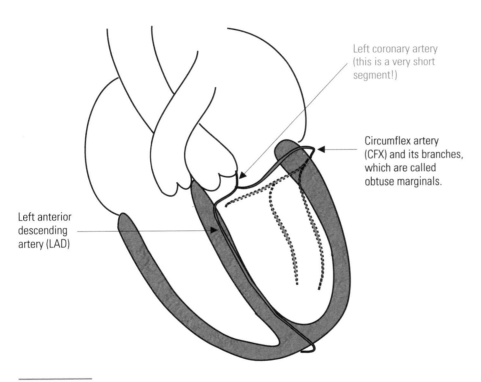

Left coronary artery (this is a very short segment!)

Circumflex artery (CFX) and its branches, which are called obtuse marginals.

Left anterior descending artery (LAD)

FIGURE 1.10

The Left Anterior Descending Artery

The LAD artery perfuses the anterior wall of the left ventricle, the anterior section of the ventricular septum, and the lateral wall of the left ventricle.

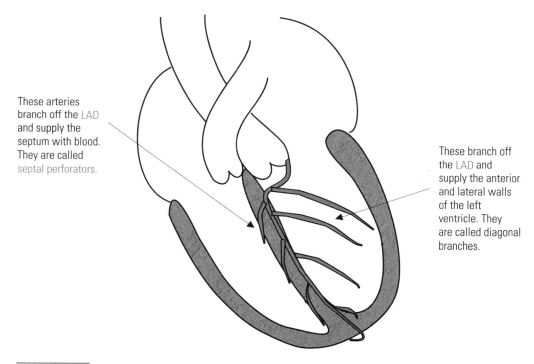

These arteries branch off the LAD and supply the septum with blood. They are called septal perforators.

These branch off the LAD and supply the anterior and lateral walls of the left ventricle. They are called diagonal branches.

FIGURE 1.11

The Circumflex Artery

The CFX branch of the left coronary artery supplies blood to the left atrium and the posterior and lateral walls of the left ventricle.

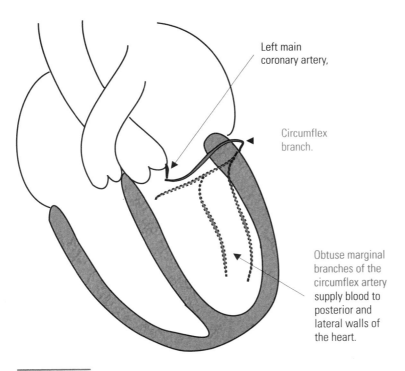

Left main coronary artery,

Circumflex branch.

Obtuse marginal branches of the circumflex artery supply blood to posterior and lateral walls of the heart.

FIGURE 1.12

Coronary Arteries as End Arteries

The three main branches of the coronary arteries typically do not connect or anastomose with each other at their ends and are therefore called "end arteries." This anatomical feature poses significant problems when atherosclerotic lesions develop in the arteries, because there is no alternate route for the blood to travel. This leads to ischemia and necrosis of the myocardial tissue.

Although the main coronary arteries are end arteries and do not connect with each other, the smaller arterial vessels can sometimes anastomose to some degree, providing what is known as collateral circulation. If collateral circulation develops, it provides a means of supplying blood to the ischemic areas of the heart. Therefore, the factors surrounding the development of collateral circulation are of great significance in the study and treatment of coronary artery disease.

FIGURE 1.13A

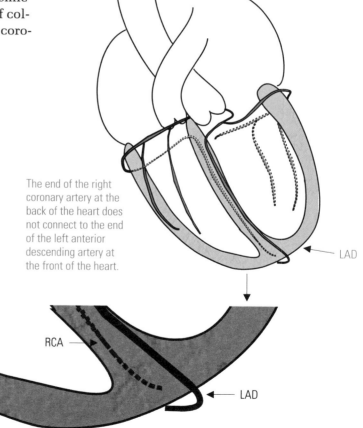

The end of the right coronary artery at the back of the heart does not connect to the end of the left anterior descending artery at the front of the heart.

LAD

FIGURE 1.13B

RCA

LAD

Blood Supply to the Myocardium

The coronary arteries lie on the outermost layer of the heart, or epicardium, and penetrate in toward the myocardium. The portion of myocardium furthest from the artery lies near the endocardium and is called subendocardial tissue. It has the poorest blood supply of the entire myocardium.

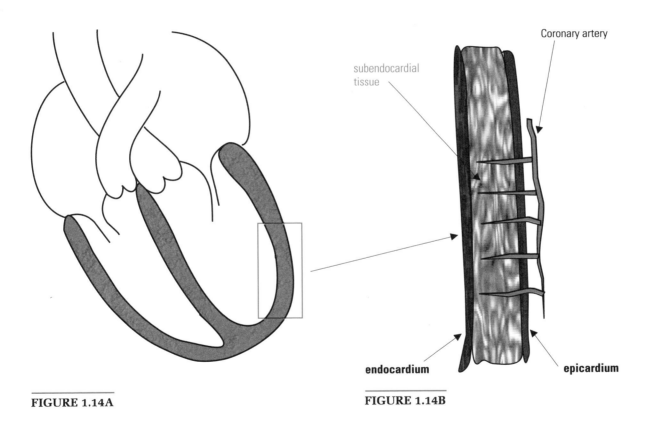

subendocardial tissue

Coronary artery

endocardium

epicardium

FIGURE 1.14A   **FIGURE 1.14B**

Physiology Review of the Heart's Conduction System

In 1913, Wilhelm Einthoven contributed significantly to the study of the heart by inventing the electrocardiogram (EKG). Einthoven attached wires or electrodes to the right arm, left arm, and left leg. This formed a theoretical triangle. When the electrodes were connected to a galvanometer, they measured the electrical activity generated within the heart. This activity, which was then recorded on paper, was representative of individual heartbeats.

Modern EKG machines inscribe 12 leads (or views) from differing combinations of the four limb electrodes and six chest wall electrodes.

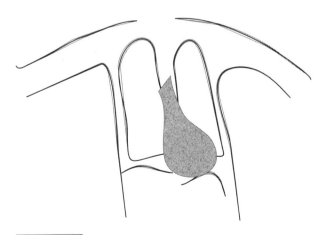

FIGURE 2.1

Self-Study Objectives

■ **Identify and describe the following:**

The six limb leads

The six precordial leads

The time lines on EKG paper

A 0.04 second time interval

A 0.20 second time interval

The EKG baseline

A positive wave

A negative wave

Measurement of wave amplitude

Standardization of the EKG

17

The 12 EKG Leads

A total of 12 leads, or views, are represented on the modern EKG. The 12 leads are consistently arranged in a standard pattern. The first six leads represent the frontal plane (or view) of the heart. They are called the limb leads and are named I, II, III, AVR, AVL, and AVL. The next six leads represent the horizontal plane (or view) of the heart. They are called precordial (in front of the heart) leads, and are named V1, V2, V3, V4, V5, and V6.

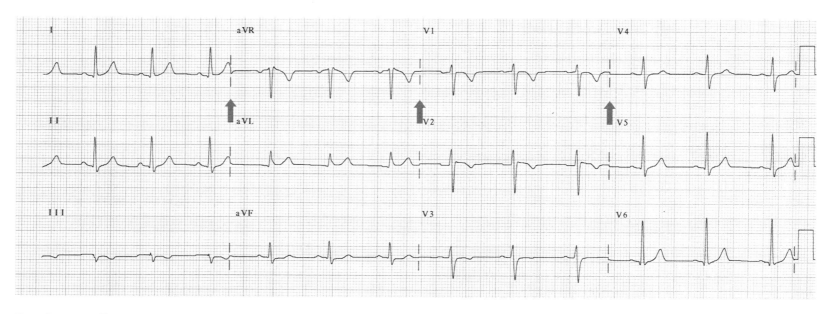

Sometimes an artifact appears where the leads change on the paper (the red arrows). It has no medical meaning, and simply signals that the EKG machine has changed the lead that it is recording.

FIGURE 2.2

EKG Paper and Time Lines

The EKG is recorded on special standardized paper that scrolls out of the machine at a specific and controlled speed. Each large box is 5mm wide and represents 0.20 seconds. Each large box is equivalent to 5 smaller 1-mm boxes, each representing 0.04 seconds. Measuring the width of any wave or interval from left to right, using the boxes as a scale, determines the duration of that wave in seconds. The normal EKG recording contains a P wave, a QRS complex, and a T wave.

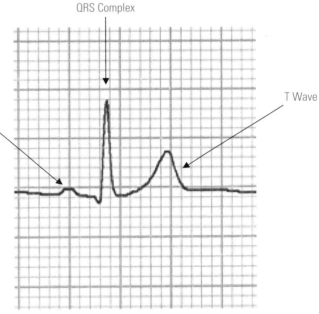

FIGURE 2.3A

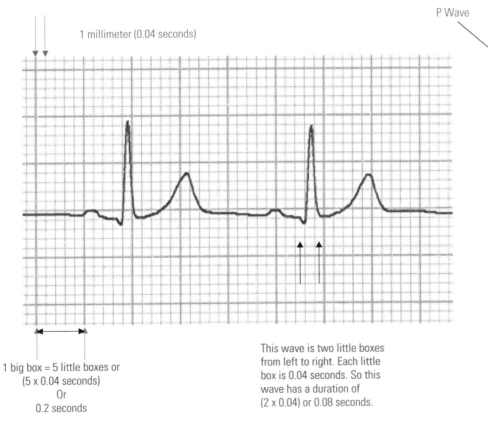

1 millimeter (0.04 seconds)

1 big box = 5 little boxes or
(5 x 0.04 seconds)
Or
0.2 seconds

This wave is two little boxes
from left to right. Each little
box is 0.04 seconds. So this
wave has a duration of
(2 x 0.04) or 0.08 seconds.

FIGURE 2.3B

The Baseline

The baseline on a 12-lead EKG is an imaginary line that connects the end of the T wave to the beginning of the P wave. All measurements of other waves are made relative to the baseline.

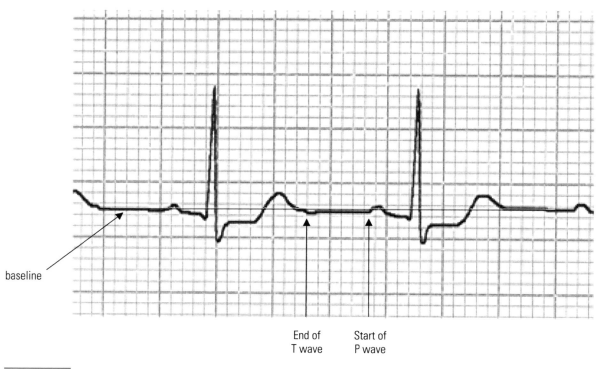

baseline

End of   Start of
T wave   P wave

FIGURE 2.4

How to Measure Waves on the EKG

Each little box is 1 mm tall (vertically). A wave that goes upward from the baseline is said to be positive. A wave that goes downward from the baseline is said to be negative. Measuring the distance of a positive wave's peak from the baseline gives the amplitude (height) of the wave in millimeters. Measuring the distance of a negative wave's lowest point from the baseline gives the amplitude (depth) of the wave in millimeters.

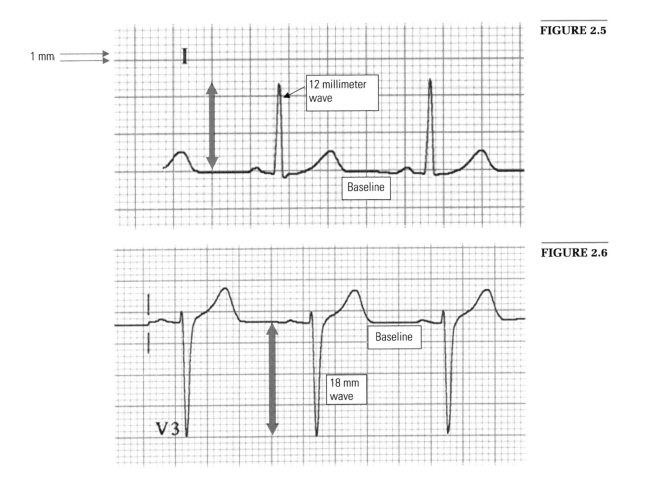

FIGURE 2.5

1 mm

I

12 millimeter wave

Baseline

FIGURE 2.6

Baseline

18 mm wave

V3

Standardization

To ensure that the EKG correctly measures and records the amplitude of waves above and below the baseline, a standardized voltage is inscribed on every EKG, usually at the right side of the EKG. It should measure exactly 10 little boxes in height.

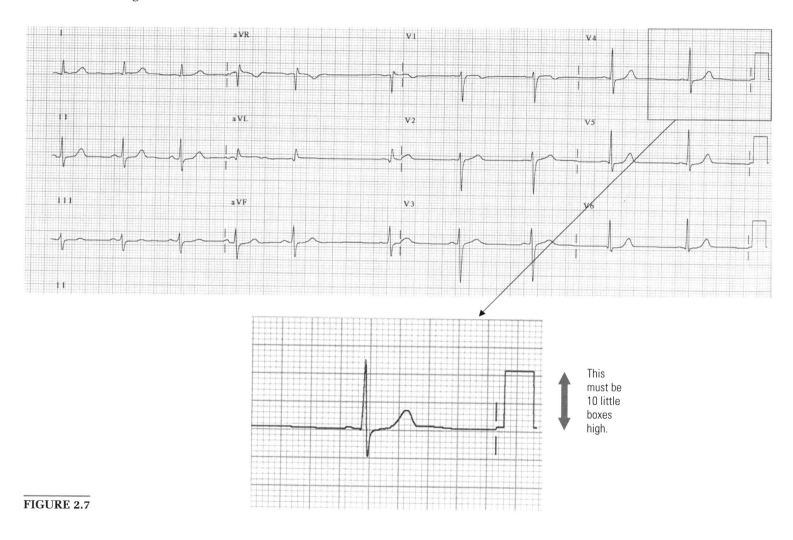

This must be 10 little boxes high.

FIGURE 2.7

Basics of the 12-Lead EKG

3

Self-Study Objectives

■ **Identify and describe the following:**

Five critical electrical and mechanical functions

Five parts of the heart's electrical system

SA node

P wave

AV node

Bundle of His

Right and left bundle branches

Purkinje fibers

QRS complex

The heart has an intricate electrical system, made up of highly specialized cells, that is responsible for generating each heart beat. The specialized cells are responsible for five critical electrical and mechanical functions: (1) establishing the ability to create an automatic and regular heart rhythm; (2) allowing communication among the billions of cells in less than one-tenth or two-tenths of a second; (3) providing for activation of the myocardial cells; (4) triggering mechanical contraction; and (5) resetting the system for the next cycle in a process called repolarization. Except for mechanical contraction, all of these functions are represented on the EKG.

The heart's electrical system consists of five structures: the sinoatrial (or SA) node, the atrioventricular (or AV) node, the bundle of His, the right and left bundle branches, and the Purkinje fibers. The right and left atria contract in atrial systole, as the electrical impulse triggers atrial contraction. The right and left ventricles contract in ventricular systole, as the electrical impulse triggers mechanical contraction (Figure 3.1).

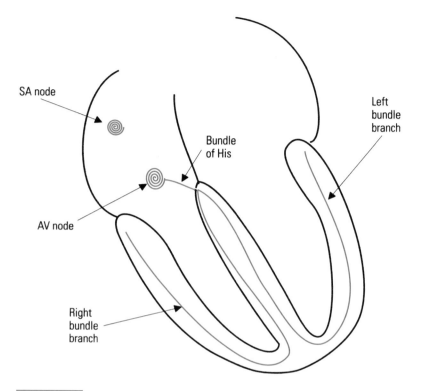

FIGURE 3.1

Creation of the Rhythm:
The Sinus Node

The sinoatrial node (SA node) is the heart's natural pacemaker because it
normally initiates each heartbeat and maintains the rest of the heart's pace.
The SA node comprises hundreds of specialized cells and is located in the
upper part of the right atrium. The SA node normally generates an average
of 60 to 100 impulses per minute. These impulses that travel through the
atria via the internodal conduction pathway cause the atria to contract. This

depolarizes both atria, as the signal also heads for the AV node (Figure 3.2). This electrical activation of the atria (called depolarization) is represented on the EKG as a "P" wave. This is normally the first wave, or "deflection," on the EKG.

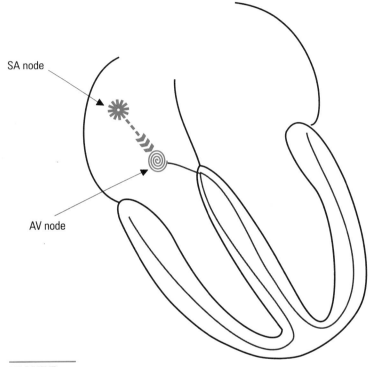

SA node

AV node

FIGURE 3.2

P waves

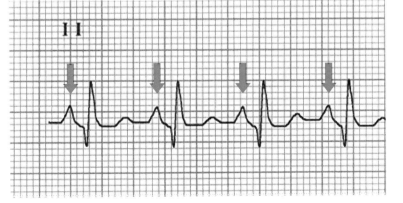

II

FIGURE 3.3

Identifying the P Wave on the EKG

Since the normal orderly process begins when the SA node depolarizes the right and left atria, we look for and see the P wave first. The size, shape, and amplitude of the P wave may vary. It may occasionally be small and difficult to find. The P wave may be mostly below the baseline (as in Figure 3.4), mostly above the baseline (as in Figure 3.5 below), or mixed. The P wave may be relatively tiny and difficult to see (as in Figure 3.6). The apparent absence of a P wave is abnormal and suggests that the rhythm may be originating form an ectopic pacemaker in the atrial wall, or in the atrioventricular junction. (See Section III for more on this subject.)

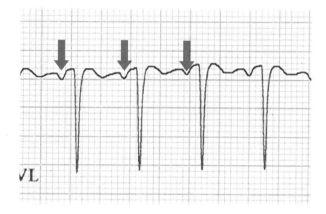

FIGURE 3.4

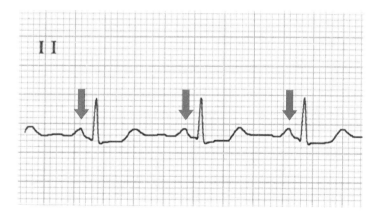

FIGURE 3.5

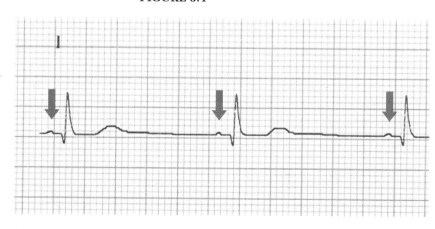

FIGURE 3.6

Communication with the Ventricles: The Atrioventricular Node and the Bundle Branches

The atrioventricular node (AV node) is located in the lower part of the right atrium. The AV node receives the impulse from the SA node and continues transmitting (communicating) it to the bundle of His.

The bundle of His is found below the AV node and communicates (conducts) the electrical impulse through to the bundle branches. The bundle branches divide into the right bundle branch, which leads to the right ventricle, and the left bundle branch, which leads to the left ventricle. The electrical stimulus travels down the bundle branches to the Purkinje fibers. Finally the myocardial cells contract, a mechanical event that is known as ventricular systole. For a detailed discussion of normal and abnormal conduction, see Chapters 9 to 12.

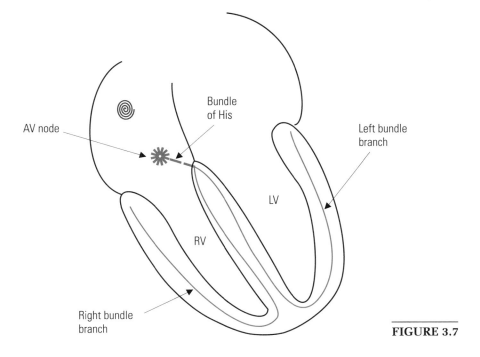

AV node

Bundle of His

Left bundle branch

LV

RV

Right bundle branch

FIGURE 3.7

Depolarization of the Ventricles:
The QRS Complex

Once the impulse reaches the Purkinje network, it spreads (communicates) onward and activates, or depolarizes, the myocardial cells. This is referred to as ventricular depolarization. Ventricular depolarization is represented on the EKG as the QRS complex.

The QRS complex is the second deflection on the normal EKG. The QRS complex consists of a Q wave, an R wave, and/or an S wave, occurring either singly or in any combination. Although the complex is called the QRS complex, it does not always contain a Q wave, an R wave, and an S wave. If the *first wave* of the complex is a downward deflection, as in Figure 3.8, the complex is considered to have a Q wave. The next upward wave is called an R wave. If the first wave of the QRS is upward, as in Figure 3.9, then this wave is called an R wave. The downward wave that follows is an S wave. Note that although the EKG in Figure 3.9 does not contain a Q wave, the whole complex is still called a QRS! When no R wave is present at all, as in Figure 3.10, these deflections are called QS waves. Finally, a QRS can have all three waves, as in Figure 3.11.

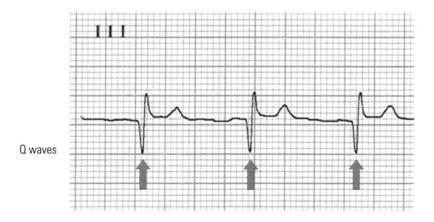

FIGURE 3.8

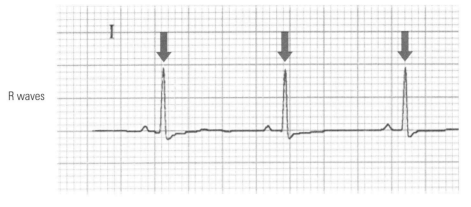

R waves

FIGURE 3.9

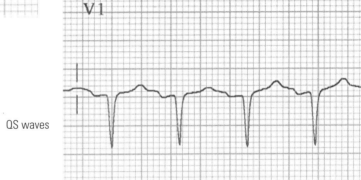

QS waves

FIGURE 3.10

QRS complex

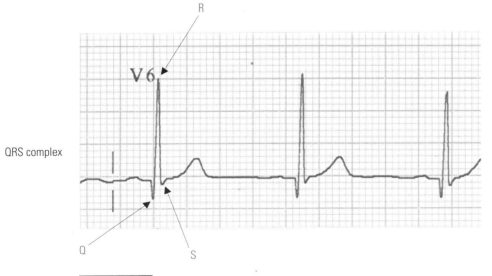

FIGURE 3.11

Repolarization of the Ventricles: The T Wave

The third deflection on the EKG is the T wave. The T wave represents ventricular repolarization. The ventricles must repolarize or recharge themselves before the next cardiac cycle can begin.

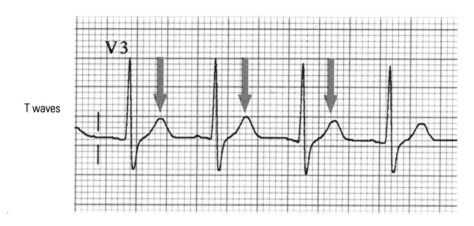

FIGURE 3.12

Methodology: Measurements and Their Clinical Significance

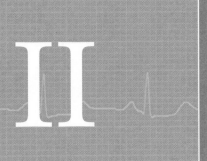

II

Heart Rate

The Heart Rate: A Mandatory Part of an EKG Interpretation

The EKG provides a skilled reader with a wealth of information about the heart. One of the most basic yet important pieces of information the EKG provides is the heart rate (HR). The heart rate is defined as the number of times the heart beats per minute. It is a vital sign. It is always clinically relevant. Calculating the heart rate is easy because the EKG is always recorded on graph paper that measures time as it travels horizontally through the machine. Ignoring the heart rate on an EKG is the single most common mistake in learning to read an EKG!

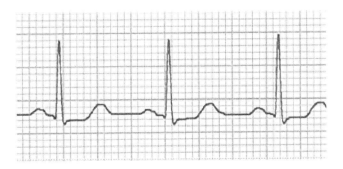

FIGURE 4.1

Measurement of the Heart Rate

The most accurate way to measure heart rate is by measuring the R-R interval. The R-R interval is the distance from one R wave to the next R wave. When measuring the R-R interval, take the beginning of one QRS complex, and count the number of "little boxes" up to the beginning of the next QRS complex. Divide this number into 1500. This method of calculating the heart rate is valid if the heart rate is regular. Table 4.1 at the end of this chapter offers a convenient method for obtaining the heart rate without doing the calculations. It is a good idea to carry such a table in your pocket for quick reference and accurate determination of the heart rate.

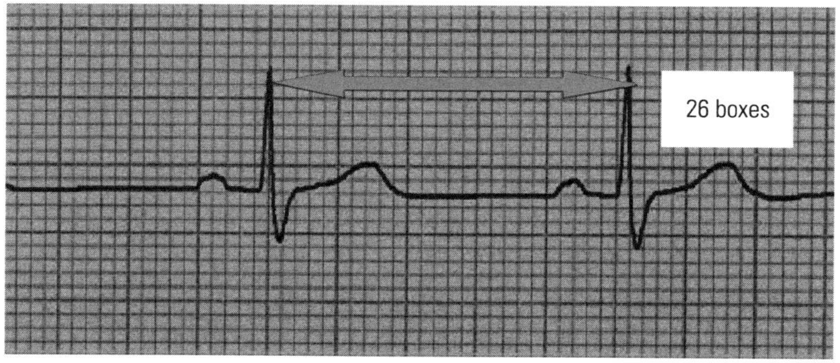

1500/26 = 58

Heart rate = 58 beats per minute

Sinus Bradycardia

26 boxes

FIGURE 4.2

The Sinus Rhythms

The sinus node normally sets and controls the heart at a rate of 60 to 100 beats per minute (bpm). **This is called sinus rhythm, or normal sinus rhythm (Figure 4.3, rate 65 bpm).** When the sinus rate is below 60 bpm, the rhythm is called sinus bradycardia **(Figure 4.4, rate 58).** When the sinus rate is greater than 100 bpm, it is called sinus tachycardia **(Figure 4.5, rate 125 bpm). The upper limit for sinus tachycardia in a given patient is estimated by a formula: (Max HR = 220 − patient's age in years). Thus, the maximum HR a person can achieve decreases with age. Sinus rhythms, regardless of rate, are typically regular. When the heart rate varies by more than 10%, the rhythm is called sinus arrhythmia.**

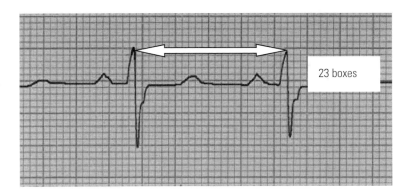

FIGURE 4.3

23 boxes

1500/23 = 65

Heart rate = 65 beats/minute

Sinus Rhythm

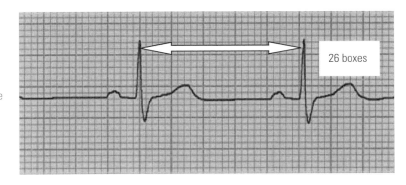

FIGURE 4.4

26 boxes

1500/26 = 58

Heart rate = 58 beats/minute

Sinus Bradycardia

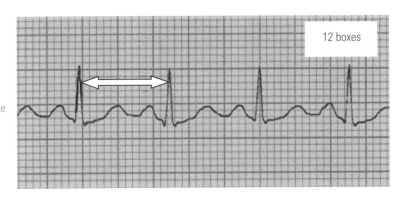

FIGURE 4.5

12 boxes

1500/12 = 125

Heart rate = 125 beats/minute

Sinus Tachycardia

The Sinus Node: Master and Servant

The sinus node normally sets and controls the rate of depolarization and contraction of the rest of the heart. In this sense, the sinus node is the master of the heart. Yet, the sinus node is itself under the control of two parts of the nervous system – the sympathetic and parasympathetic nervous systems. These two forces are always active, with either one able to predominate depending on the clinical situation.

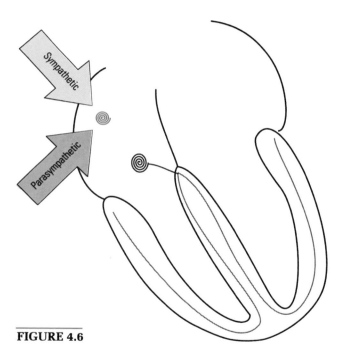

FIGURE 4.6

Sinus Tachycardia: Pathophysiology (Critical Concept!)

Sinus tachycardia represents a relative imbalance in the normal sympathetic/parasympathetic balance of the heart. There are two basic causes of sinus tachycardia: (1) increased sympathetic activity or (2) decreased parasympathetic activity. **Increased sympathetic activity is by far more common clinically. Increased sympathetic activity is part of the ancient "flight or fight" protective emergency system of the body. It is analogous to someone inside the patient's body calling a "code" or pulling a fire alarm. It is that serious, and that significant. The underlying cause should always be determined. It will typically be very relevant clinically.** Causes of increased sympathetic activity include shock, heart failure, infection, bleeding, pain, pulmonary

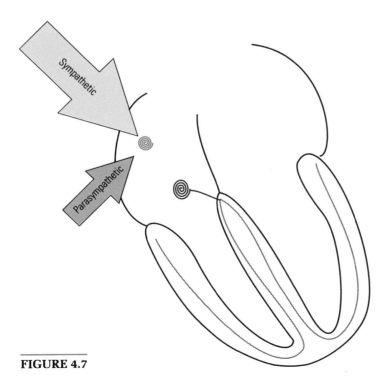

FIGURE 4.7

embolism, hypoxia, hypoglycemia, anxiety, and drugs. All are major disorders. Commonly used drugs that cause increased sympathetic activity include bronchodilators, inotropic infusions, and pressors. From the EKG, diagnose sinus tachycardia, and then evaluate the patient to determine its cause. Decreased parasympathetic activity is a much less common cause of sinus tachycardia and is most commonly related to atropine administration or poison ingestion. THE MOST COMMON BIG MISTAKE EKG READERS MAKE IS IGNORING THE PRESENCE OF SINUS TACHYCARDIA. A return to the bedside frequently provides the answer!

Sinus Tachycardia: Clinically Based Critical Thinking

The finding of sinus tachycardia on the EKG, as in Figure 4.8, enables visualization of an imbalance in the normal sympathetic/parasympathetic balance. Underlying clinical possibilities should be considered. The sympathetic stimulation may have increased, or the parasympathetic stimulation may have decreased (Figure 4.9).

For example, the ER admission of a patient with an acute MI and sinus tachycardia can have several causes. Shock, congestive heart failure, pain, anxiety, hypoxia and bleeding (secondary to anticoagulation) may be present singly or in combination. The vital signs document the blood pressure and heart rate. Physical examination of the lungs for rales helps to confirm the presence of congestive heart failure. Pulse oximetry, if available, confirms the presence or absence of hypoxemia. The CXR helps to confirm CHF, or a pneumothorax. An echocardiogram determines systolic and diastolic function, as well as the presence or absence of mechanical complications of acute MI. This is clinically oriented critical thinking. It all begins with the heart rate, a vital sign, right there on the EKG!

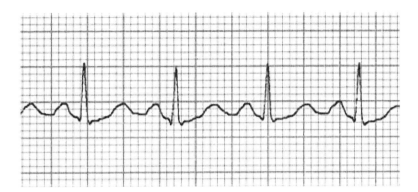

FIGURE 4.8

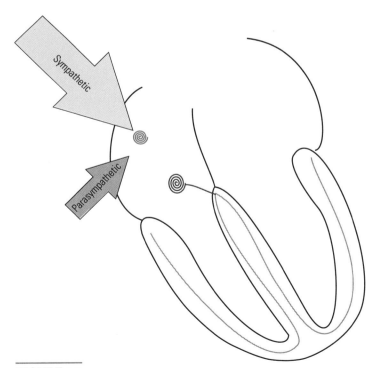

FIGURE 4.9

Sinus Bradycardia: Pathophysiology

Sinus bradycardia represents a relative imbalance in the normal sympathetic/ parasympathetic balance of the heart. There are two basic causes of sinus bradycardia: (1) decreased sympathetic activity or (2) increased parasympathetic activity. Parasympathetic activity is frequently the "relax and take your time" signal that counterbalances the sympathetic nervous system. Increasing parasympathetic activity slows down the heart rate. Decreased sympathetic activity does the same and is more common clinically. It is the result of the current common practice of using drugs that block the sympathetic nervous system in the treatment of hypertension, coronary artery disease, and heart failure. It is also possible to directly stimulate the parasympathetic nervous system. A common cause of increased parasympathetic activity is the vagal response. The vagal response can occur secondary to gastrointestinal (GI) stimulation during nausea and vomiting, drug treatment, the carotid reflex, or with direct therapeutic vagal stimulation for seizures or depression.

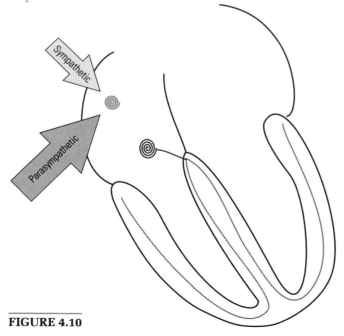

FIGURE 4.10

The Heart Rate in Atrial Fibrillation

When the RR intervals are irregular, the best way to estimate the heart rate is by counting the number of QRS complexes in a 6-second block of time and multiplying that number by 10. (Five large boxes measure one second of time. Thirty large boxes measure 6 seconds of time.) The result is the heart rate in beats per minute. In the example below, there are 7 QRS complexes in the 6-second block. Multiplying 7 complexes (in 6 seconds) by 10 yields a heart rate of 70 per minute. Of course, since the rhythm is atrial fibrillation, this rate of 70 represents the ventricular rate.

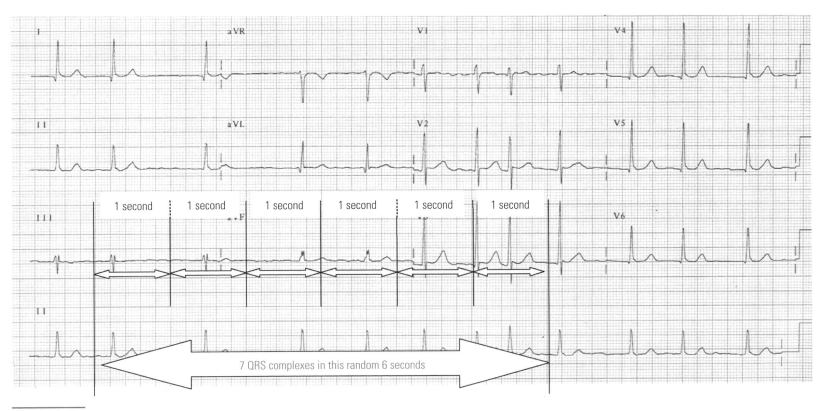

FIGURE 4.11

The Heart Rate Reference Table

Table 4.1 provides a quick reference for accurate determination of the heart rate when the patient is in a regular rhythm.

TABLE 4.1 **Table of Heart Rates**

Number of Little Boxes	Heart Rate	Number of Little Boxes	Heart Rate	Number of Little Boxes	Heart Rate
5	300	18	83	31	48
6	250	19	79	32	47
7	214	20	75	33	45
8	188	21	71	34	44
9	167	22	68	35	43
10	150	23	65	36	42
11	136	24	63	37	41
12	125	25	60	38	39
13	115	26	58	39	38
14	107	27	56	40	38
15	100	28	54	41	37
16	94	29	52	42	36
17	88	30	50	43	35

Clinical Significance of Heart Rates: Summary

The heart rate is a vital sign and conveys critical information.
Some causes of sinus tachycardia:

- Shock
- Heart failure
- Bleeding
- Infection
- Hyperthyroidism
- Pulmonary embolism
- Sympathomimetic drug therapy
- Anxiety
- Hypoglycemia
- Hypoxia

Some causes of sinus bradycardia:

- Beta blocker therapy
- Vagal response (increased parasympathetic tone)
- Hypothyroidism
- Athlete's conditioning

CHAPTER 4 WORKSHEETS

SAMPLE COMPLETED WORKSHEET

BASIC MEASUREMENTS		
Parameter	Measurement	Interpretation
HR	136	Abnormal
Rhythm	Sinus tach	Abnormal
PR		
QRS		
QT		
QTc		
P direction		
QRS direction		

Instructions for Chapter 4 Worksheets

A) Count the number of small boxes between two QRS complexes. Divide that number into 1500 to accurately determine the HR.
B) Use the heart rate to classify the rhythm as sinus rhythm (60 to 100), sinus tachycardia (greater than 100), or sinus bradycardia (less than 60).
C) Provide an interpretation

Clinically Based Critical Thinking: Interpretation

Sinus tachycardia should always be evaluated and explained clinically. It is a vital sign, and always has clinical relevance. Relative predominance of the sympathetic nervous system or relative inhibition of the parasympathetic nervous system typically causes sinus tachycardia.

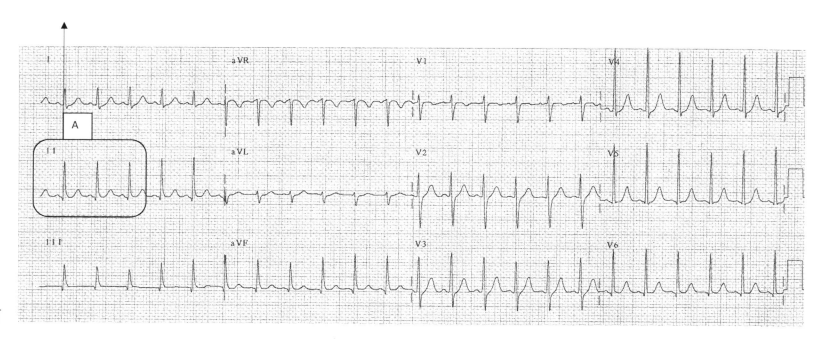

FIGURE 4.12

BASIC MEASUREMENTS

Parameter	Measurement	Interpretation
HR		
Rhythm		
PR		
QRS		
QT		
QTc		
P direction		
QRS direction		

Instructions for Chapter 4 Worksheets

A) Count the number of small boxes between two QRS complexes. Divide that number into 1500 to accurately determine the HR.
B) Use the heart rate to classify the rhythm as sinus rhythm (60 to 100), sinus tachycardia (greater than 100), or sinus bradycardia (less than 60).
C) Provide an interpretation

Clinically Based Critical Thinking: Interpretation

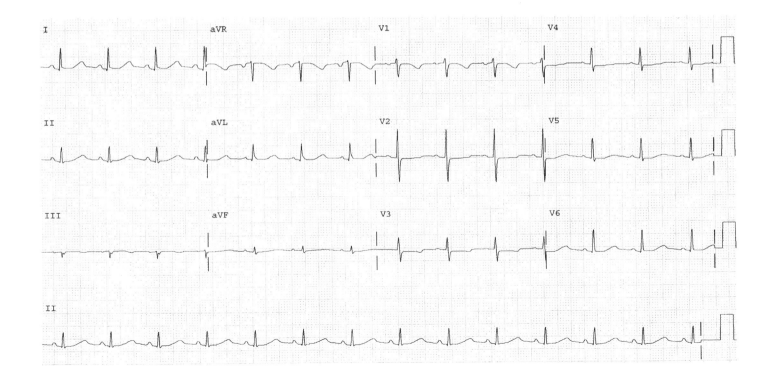

WORKSHEET 4.2

BASIC MEASUREMENTS		
Parameter	Measurement	Interpretation
HR		
Rhythm		
PR		
QRS		
QT		
QTc		
P direction		
QRS direction		

Instructions for Chapter 4 Worksheets

A) Count the number of small boxes between two QRS complexes. Divide that number into 1500 to accurately determine the HR.
B) Use the heart rate to classify the rhythm as sinus rhythm (60 to 100), sinus tachycardia (greater than 100), or sinus bradycardia (less than 60).
C) Provide an interpretation

Clinically Based Critical Thinking: Interpretation

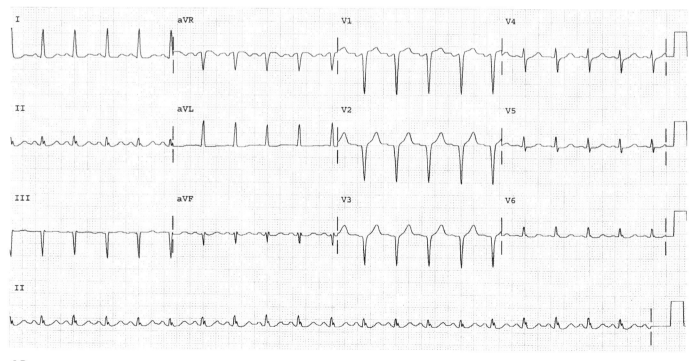

BASIC MEASUREMENTS

Parameter	Measurement	Interpretation
HR		
Rhythm		
PR		
QRS		
QT		
QTc		
P direction		
QRS direction		

Instructions for Chapter 4 Worksheets

A) Count the number of small boxes between two QRS complexes. Divide that number into 1500 to accurately determine the HR.
B) Use the heart rate to classify the rhythm as sinus rhythm (60 to 100), sinus tachycardia (greater than 100), or sinus bradycardia (less than 60).
C) Provide an interpretation

Clinically Based Critical Thinking: Interpretation

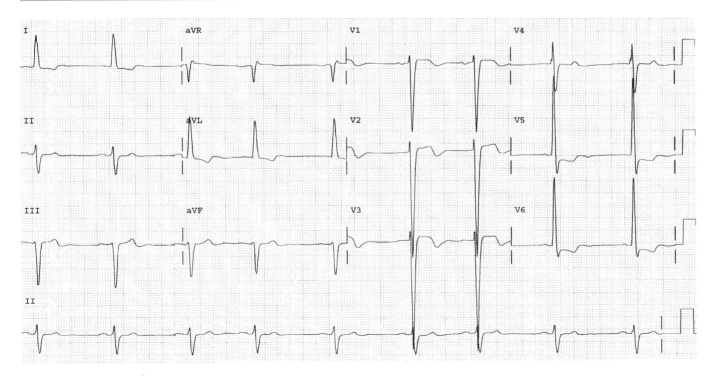

The PR, QRS, and QT Intervals

The PR, QRS, and QT Intervals

After calculation of the the heart rate, the next step is to measure the **PR, QRS, and QT intervals.** These are not optional measurements! Like heart rate, the intervals are measured left to right in **units of time** (seconds). The lighter vertical lines on the EKG are time lines that are 0.04 seconds (or one "little box") apart (see Figure 5.1). The darker vertical lines are 0.2 seconds (or one

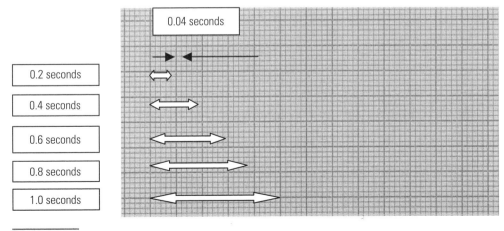

0.04 seconds
0.2 seconds
0.4 seconds
0.6 seconds
0.8 seconds
1.0 seconds

FIGURE 5.1

"big box") apart. One big box contains 5 little boxes and is (5 times 0.04) or 0.2 seconds. The PR, QRS, and QT intervals are measured on all EKGs. They are measured only in the limb leads. The limb leads (I, II, III, AVR, AVL, and AVF) are also called the frontal plane leads (see Figure 5.2). These intervals are never measured in the precordial or horizontal plane leads (V1, V2, V3, V4, V5, and V6).

Frontal plane   Limb leads (I, II, III, AVR, AVL, AVF)

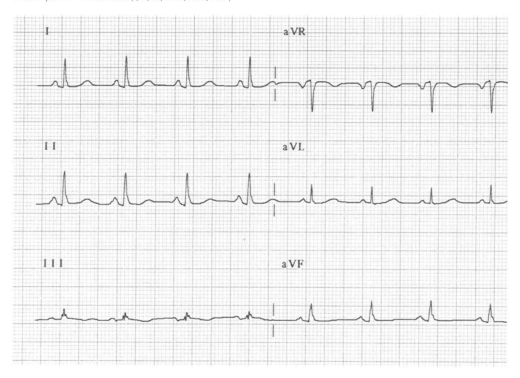

FIGURE 5.2

The Sequence of Events

The sequence of events in the cardiac cycle starts with the automatic firing of the sinus node (see Figure 5.3). The impulse passes through and depolarizes the atria. As the atrial cells depolarize, they cause the P wave to appear on the EKG. After its trip through the atria, the impulse slowly passes through the AV node. After exiting the AV node, the impulse goes through the bundle of His and the right and left bundle branches. Finally it depolarizes the ventricles, which causes the QRS to appear on the EKG.

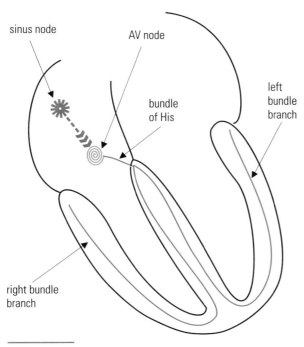

FIGURE 5.3

The PR Interval:
An Intentional Delay

The PR interval measures the duration of time from the very beginning of atrial activation to the very beginning of ventricular depolarization. The very beginning of atrial activation appears as the start of the P wave, which is where measurement of the PR interval should begin. The very beginning of ventricular activation appears as the start of the QRS, which is where the measurement of the PR interval should end. (A better name for this interval would have been the P-QRS interval!) Most of the time, the PR interval is a physiological, or intentional, delay in transmitting the activation through the AV node. This delay is very important, because it allows the atria time to contract and pump blood into the ventricles before the ventricles begin to contract with the start of the QRS. Remember, the reason for these electrical

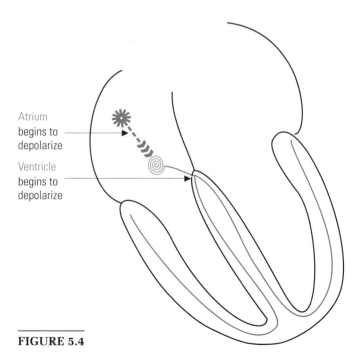

Atrium begins to depolarize

Ventricle begins to depolarize

FIGURE 5.4

events is to pump blood! Thus the atria contract, the AV node delays a bit so blood can flow into and fill the ventricles, and then the ventricles contract. Without the AV delay, the heart could not effectively pump in sequence. It would look like an assembly line gone wrong in an old *I Love Lucy* episode.

How to Measure the PR Interval

The PR interval is measured from the very beginning of the P wave to the very beginning of the QRS in the limb leads only, that is, Leads I, II, III, AVR, AFL, or AVF. In this example, the PR interval is 3.0 little boxes. Each little box represents 0.04 second. Thus, 3 boxes × 0.04 seconds per box equals 0.12 seconds. Therefore. this PR interval (3 × 0.04) is 0.12 seconds long. The normal PR interval is 0.12 seconds to 0.2 seconds. This PR interval is normal.

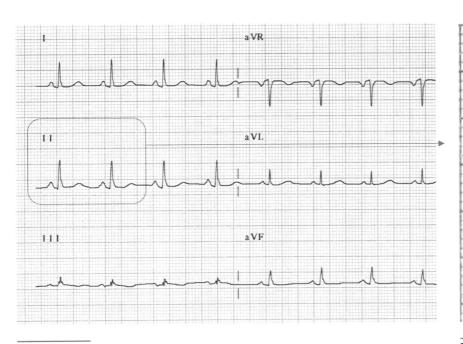

FIGURE 5.5a

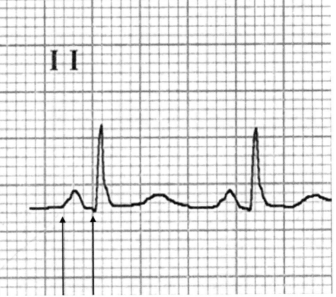

FIGURE 5.5b

Long PR Intervals: 1° Atrioventricular Block

Diseases of the AV node can prolong conduction through the AV node to greater than 0.20 seconds. This is called first-degree AV block (1° AV block). Causes of 1° AV block include coronary artery disease, drug toxicity, infectious diseases such as Lyme disease, rheumatic fever, endocarditis, and degenerative diseases. AV block can be found in trained athletes, where an increased delay is necessary to allow more blood to enter the ventricle with every heart beat. As before, measure from the very beginning of the P wave to the very beginning of the QRS in the limb leads only, that is, Leads I, II, III, AVR, AFL, or AVF. In this example, the PR interval is 9.0 boxes. Each little box represents 0.04 seconds. Thus, 9 boxes × 0.04 seconds for each box equals 0.36 seconds. Therefore, this PR interval (9 × 0.04) is 0.36 seconds long. The normal PR interval is 0.12 seconds to 0.2 seconds. This PR interval is longer than 0.20 seconds, so it is called 1° AV block.

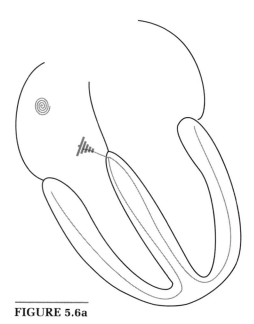

This PR interval measures 9 boxes or 0.36 seconds

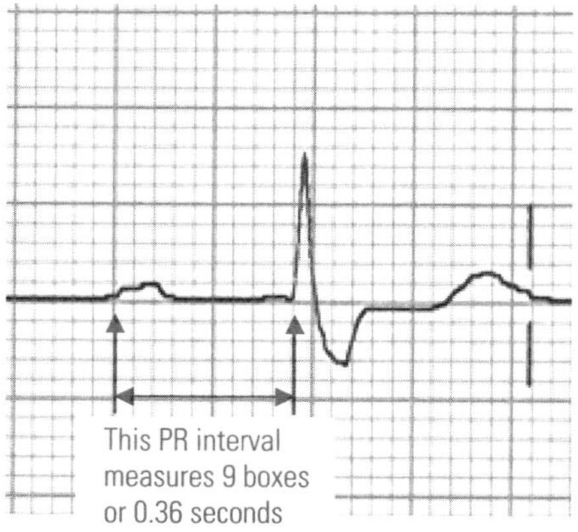

FIGURE 5.6b

FIGURE 5.6a

Short PR Interval: WPW Syndrome

Figure 5.7a demonstrates an abnormal pathway that is present in some people. This pathway connects the atria to the ventricles, bypassing the normal AV node. As a result, the PR interval is shorter than 0.12 seconds. It is abnormally short because without the normal AV delay, some part of both ventricles start to depolarize too early. This produces an early depolarization of the ventricles, called a delta wave, as shown in Figure 5.7b. This short circuit is called an AV bypass tract, short PR syndrome, or WPW syndrome (named after Drs. *Wolff*, *Parkinson*, and *White*). It can be as dangerous as it sounds and can lead to fatally fast heart rates, as shown in Figure 5.7c. Careful inspection of this rhythm strip shows that successive R waves are as close as 4 little boxes apart. This calculates to a heart rate of 1500/4 or 375 bpm! **The normal AV node has a built-in maximum allowable transmission rate to protect the ventricles.** The only way to bypass this safety mechanism is with a genetic short circuit between the atria and ventricles. The ventricles simply cannot contract at this accelerated rate. (As an experiment, try to open and close the fingers of your hand into a fist at a rate of 5 or 6 times a second. That's what the ventricles are trying to do at a rate of 300 to 360 bpm!) The ventricles cannot sustain a cardiac output at this rate, and the arrhythmia must be terminated.

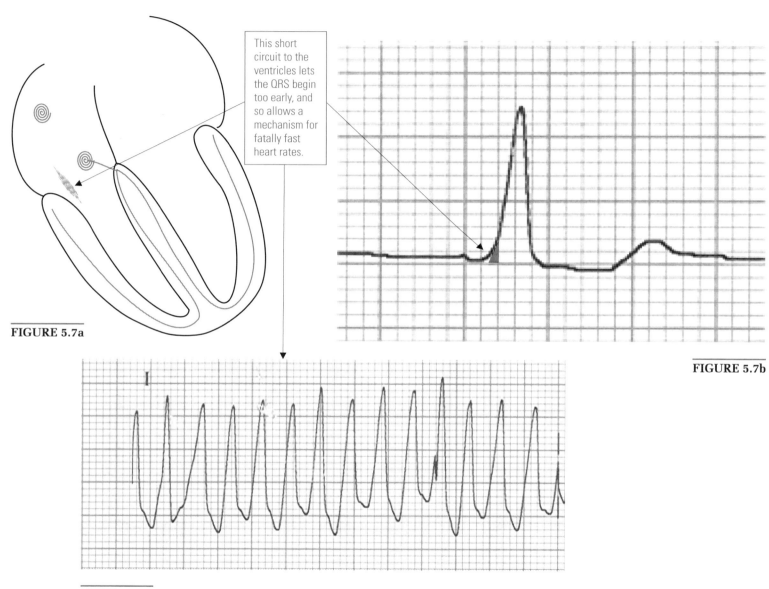

This short circuit to the ventricles lets the QRS begin too early, and so allows a mechanism for fatally fast heart rates.

FIGURE 5.7a

FIGURE 5.7b

FIGURE 5.7c

Short PR Interval: WPW Syndrome—Example

Although the PR interval is measured only in the limb leads, examination of all the leads can help in the diagnosis of WPW syndrome. Leads I and AVL demonstrate a delta wave (the slurred upstroke) at the beginning of the QRS associated with the short PR interval. Leads V1 through V6 do as well.

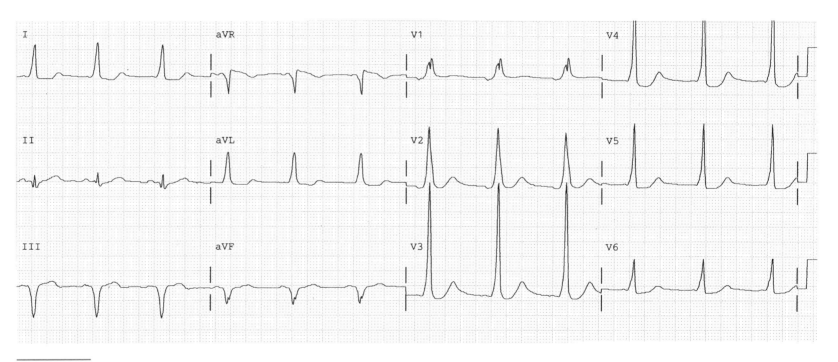

FIGURE 5.7d

Short PR Interval: WPW Syndrome and Supraventricular Tachycardia

The short circuit in WPW bypasses the normal AV node and its safety delay. If the patient develops atrial fibrillation or atrial flutter, the ventricles may be bombarded with impulses at a rate of over 300 bpm, as shown in Figure 5.7e.

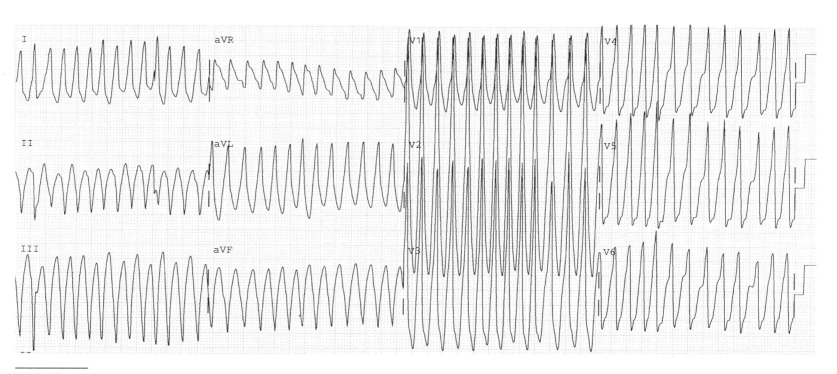

FIGURE 5.7e

The QRS Interval

The next step after measuring and analyzing the PR interval is to evaluate the QRS interval. The QRS interval measures the time from the beginning of ventricular activation, which is the beginning of the QRS (whether it is a Q or an R wave!), and the end of ventricular activation, which is the end of the QRS. The QRS interval represents the amount of time it takes for the electrical impulse to depolarize the ventricles. The normal QRS interval is 0.09 seconds or less. This means that the billions of cardiac cells that make up the ventricles are depolarized in less than 1/10 of a second. To accomplish this, a remarkable communication system relays the message from the AV node to two rapidly conducting firewires called the right bundle branch and the left bundle branch.

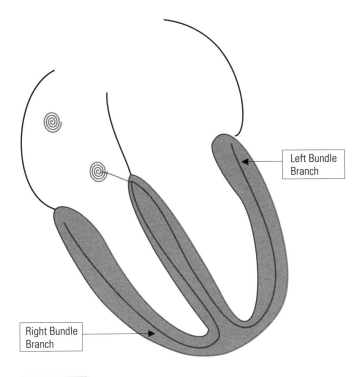

Left Bundle
Branch

Right Bundle
Branch

FIGURE 5.8

To imagine how incredible this is, picture yourself standing in front of an auditorium filled with 1,000 people (not the billions of cells in the ventricles). Ask the crowd to stand at the snap of a finger. How long would it take for everyone to get the message and begin to stand? A few seconds? In the heart, billions of cells get the message, and ALL start to stand in less than a tenth of a second!

How to Measure the QRS Interval

The QRS interval is measured from the beginning of the QRS to the end of the QRS in the limb leads only. In this example, the QRS interval is 2.0 boxes. Each little box represents 0.04 seconds. Thus, 2 boxes × 0.04 seconds for each box equals 0.08 seconds. Therefore, this QRS interval (2 × 0.04) is 0.08 seconds. Normally, the QRS interval is 0.08 to 0.09 seconds. It is normal if it is less than 0.10 seconds or less. This QRS interval is normal.

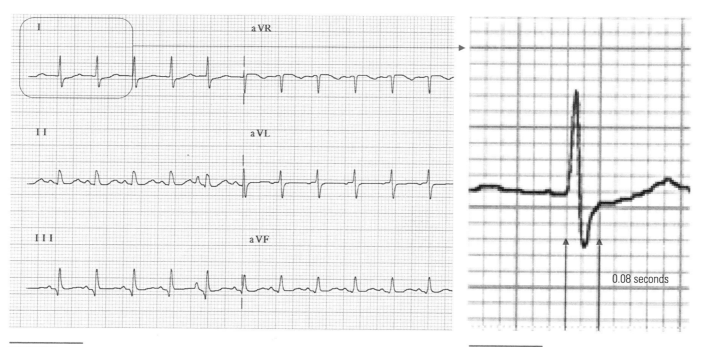

FIGURE 5.9a   **FIGURE 5.9b**

Long QRS Intervals: Intraventricular Conduction Delay and Bundle Branch Block

The normal right and left bundle branches are able to depolarize the normal right and left ventricle in less than 0.10 seconds, on average. A QRS interval of 0.10 seconds or more indicates a delay in conduction. The QRS interval in Figure 5.11 measures 2.5 little boxes, or 0.10 seconds long. A QRS interval of 0.10 second or greater (but less than 0.12 seconds) is given the awful name of IVCD. If the QRS interval reaches 0.12 seconds or longer, then bundle branch block is present. The QRS interval in Figure 5.12 is 3 little boxes wide, or 0.12 seconds long, indicating the presence of bundle branch block. Right and left bundle branch blocks will be fully discussed in Chapters 11 and 12.

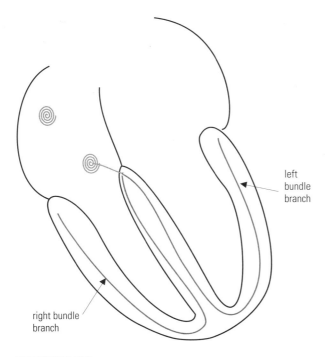

left
bundle
branch

right bundle
branch

FIGURE 5.10

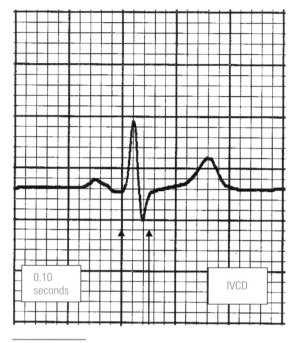

FIGURE 5.11

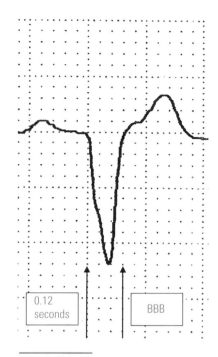

FIGURE 5.12

The QT Interval

The last interval to be measured on the EKG is the QT interval. The QT measures the distance from the beginning of the QRS to the end of the T wave. The QT represents the time it takes the ventricles to depolarize and then reset or repolarize for the next cycle. Depolarization is a relatively quick process that can be compared to releasing a stretched rubber band. Repolarization is a slower process, similar to restretching the rubber band. Depolarization and repolarization require a normal environment of oxygen and electrolytes and are very sensitive to drug effects.

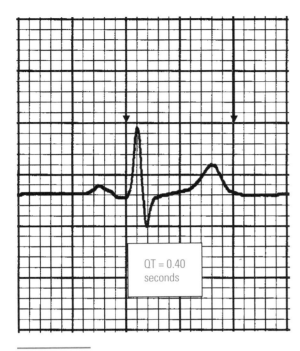

QT = 0.40
seconds

FIGURE 5.13

The QTc: QT Interval
Corrected for Heart Rate

The normal QT interval depends on the heart rate. The faster the heart rate,
the shorter the QT interval. The slower the heart rate, the longer the QT.
(If you keep releasing the rubberband faster and faster, you need to restretch
it faster and faster as well.) The QT must take into account the heart rate.
Several formulas have been proposed to correct for heart rate. Bazett's formula is the best known and most widely used. It provides the corrected QT
interval (QTc) using the heart rate and the measured QT. Normally, the QTc
is in the range of 0.365 to 0.440 seconds. This is referred to clinically as 365

or 440 milliseconds. Table 5.1 can help determine if the measured QT is normal for a given heart rate, particularly for heart rates below 100. To use the chart, first measure the heart rate and QT interval on the EKG. Then find the heart rate on the left side of the table and locate the measured QT to the right. The top of the column determines if it is normal, long, or dangerously long.

TABLE 5.1 Approximating the QT Interval

Heart Rate	Normal Range of the QT		Long QT	Dangerously Long QT
	(QTc 365)	(QTc 419)	(QTc 440)	(QTc 500)
50	0.40	0.46	0.48	0.55
55	0.38	0.44	0.46	0.52
60	0.37	0.42	0.44	0.50
65	0.35	0.40	0.42	0.48
70	0.34	0.39	0.41	0.46
75	0.33	0.37	0.39	0.45
80	0.32	0.36	0.38	0.43
85	0.31	0.35	0.37	0.42
90	0.30	0.34	0.36	0.41
95	0.29	0.33	0.35	0.40
100	0.28	0.32	0.34	0.39
105	0.28	0.32	0.33	0.38
110	0.27	0.31	0.32	0.37
115	0.26	0.30	0.32	0.36
120	0.26	0.30	0.31	0.35
125	0.25	0.29	0.30	0.35
130	0.25	0.28	0.30	0.34
135	0.24	0.28	0.29	0.33
140	0.24	0.27	0.29	0.33
145	0.23	0.27	0.28	0.32
150	0.23	0.26	0.28	0.32
155	0.23	0.26	0.27	0.31
160	0.22	0.26	0.27	0.31

Short QTc Syndrome (SQTS)

A short QT interval occurs when the QTc is shorter than it should be for the heart rate. Short QT syndome can be inherited or acquired. The inherited form has been described only recently. It is associated with specific abnormalities of the cell membrane channels, the doors in the cell membrane that let the charged ions in and out. SQTS allows potassium ions (K+) to leave the cell (through the broken door) more freely during repolarization. The cell is ready to depolarize too soon, and this predisposes to atrial fibrillation, syncope, ventricular fibrillation , and sudden death. It can occur in young healthy people with no history of heart disease. With this syndrome, the QT does not appear to decrease with increasing heart rate, but appears very short in normal heart rates, usually approximately 0.30 seconds. Because the QT normally decreases with faster heart rates, it is better to recheck the QT at rates less than 100 beats per minute. If the measured QT (before correction) is less than 0.32 seconds, then remeasure it and calculate the QTc. In this syndrome, electrophysiologic testing (EPS) directly measures and confirms the decreased refractory periods (shorter repolarization times) for both the atria and ventricles. Some drug treatments and acquired diseases can also shorten the QT and QTc. These include treatment with digitalis and hypercalcemia.

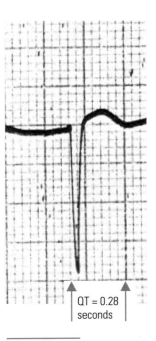

QT = 0.28 seconds

FIGURE 5.14

The Long QTc Interval

A long QT interval is present when the corrected QT interval (QTc) is greater than 0.44 seconds. The closer the QTc gets to 0.50 seconds, the more dangerous it becomes. Prolonged QTc is associated with sudden death because of malignant ventricular arrhythmias, particularly polymorphous ventricular tachycardia (torsade). Prolonged QTc can be inherited or acquired. The inherited form is termed long QT syndrome (LQTS). As with short QTc, the etiology is abnormal channels (channelopathies) on the cell membrane. These are the doors that let ions into and out of cells. In the case of long QTc, the abnormal channel function delays the cell's repolarization. This appears on the

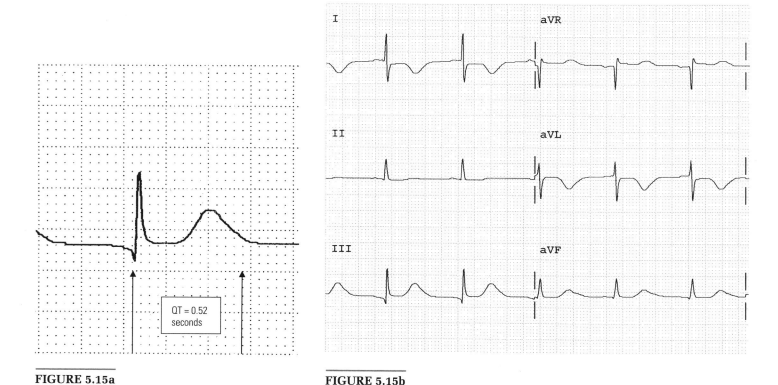

QT = 0.52 seconds

FIGURE 5.15a

FIGURE 5.15b

EKG as a long QT interval. An uncorrected QT that measures 0.40 seconds or more is probably long. A QTc greater than 0.44 seconds may be at a dangerous level. Acquired long QT syndrome is typically caused by drug effects or abnormal electrolyte imbalance.

The Indeterminate QT Interval

Sometimes, the T wave is of low amplitude and just plain hard to see. This can make a reliable measurement of the QT interval impossible. In this case, use the term "indeterminate" to describe the QT interval. As with long QT, it may be the result of drug or electrolyte effects, particularly low potassium (K^+).

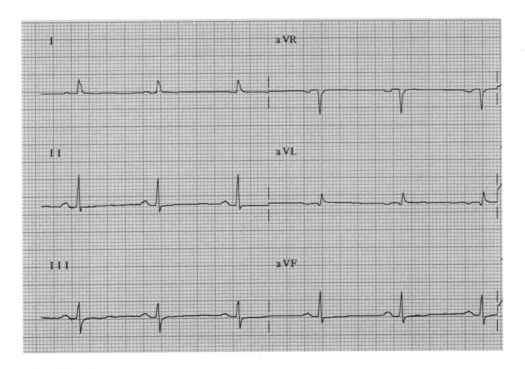

FIGURE 5.16

SAMPLE COMPLETED WORKSHEET

BASIC MEASUREMENTS

Parameter	Measurement	Interpretation
HR	115	Abnormal
Rhythm	Sinus tach	Abnormal
PR	0.14	Normal
QRS	0.08	Normal
QT	0.36	
QTc	0.50	Long
P direction		
QRS direction		

Instructions for Chapter 5 Worksheets

A) Complete basic measurements.
B) Measure the PR, QRS, and QT intervals. Interpret the PR as normal, short, or long. Interpret the QRS as normal (0.09 seconds or less), IVCD (0.10 to 0.11), or BBB (0.12 seconds or more). Assess the QT interval against the HR/QTc chart to estimate normal, long, or short QTc.
C) Provide an interpretation.

Clinically Based Critical Thinking: Interpretation

Sinus tachycardia should always be evaluated and explained clinically. Long QTc is present and commonly due to drug toxicity or electrolyte abnormalities. Hypokalemia or hypocalcemia would be common causes and should be evaluated clinically. This patient's K⁺ was 3.1. The combination of sinus tachycardia and long QTc suggests the possibility of hypovolemia and hypokalemia due to diuresis, or hypovolemia and hypocalcemia secondary to multiple transfusions.

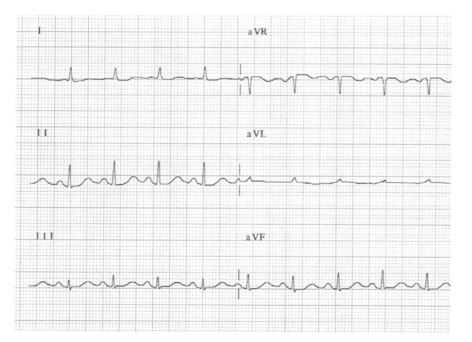

FIGURE 5.17a

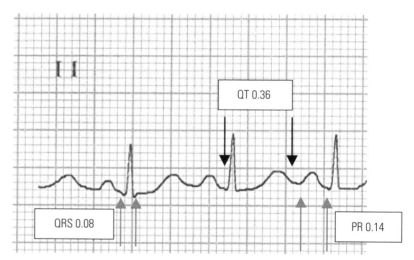

QT 0.36

QRS 0.08

PR 0.14

FIGURE 5.17b

BASIC MEASUREMENTS

Parameter	Measurement	Interpretation
HR		
Rhythm		
PR		
QRS		
QT		
QTc		
P direction		
QRS direction		

Instructions for Chapter 5 Worksheets

A) Complete basic measurements.
B) Measure the PR, QRS, and QT intervals. Interpret the PR as normal, short, or long. Interpret the QRS as normal (0.09 seconds or less), IVCD (0.10 to 0.11), or BBB (0.12 seconds or more). Assess the QT interval against the HR/QTc chart to estimate normal, long, or short QTc.
C) Provide an interpretation.

Clinically Based Critical Thinking: Interpretation

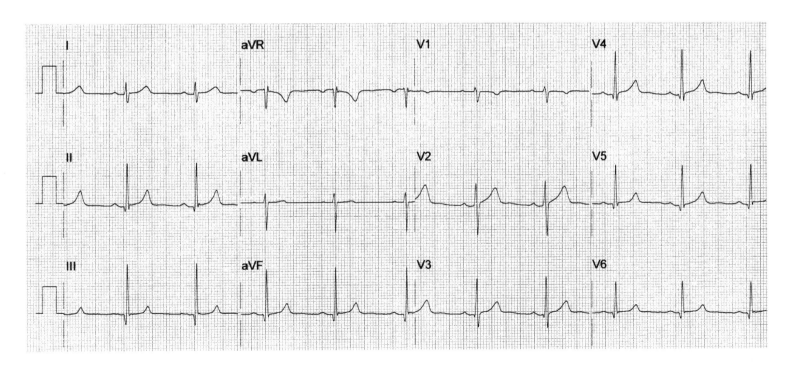

WORKSHEET 5.2

BASIC MEASUREMENTS		
Parameter	Measurement	Interpretation
HR		
Rhythm		
PR		
QRS		
QT		
QTc		
P direction		
QRS direction		

Instructions for Chapter 5 Worksheets

A) Complete basic measurements.
B) Measure the PR, QRS, and QT intervals. Interpret the PR as normal, short, or long. Interpret the QRS as normal (0.09 seconds or less), IVCD (0.10 to 0.11), or BBB (0.12 seconds or more). Assess the QT interval against the HR/QTc chart to estimate normal, long, or short QTc.
C) Provide an interpretation.

Clinically Based Critical Thinking: Interpretation

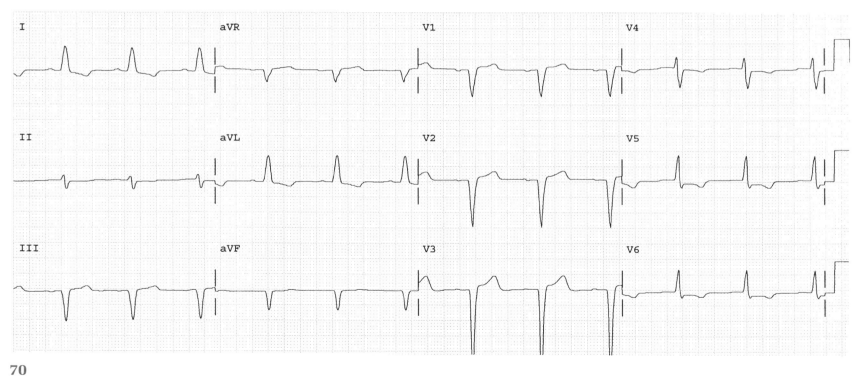

BASIC MEASUREMENTS		
Parameter	Measurement	Interpretation
HR		
Rhythm		
PR		
QRS		
QT		
QTc		
P direction		
QRS direction		

Instructions for Chapter 5 Worksheets

A) Complete basic measurements.
B) Measure the PR, QRS, and QT intervals. Interpret the PR as normal, short, or long. Interpret the QRS as normal (0.09 seconds or less), IVCD (0.10 to 0.11), or BBB (0.12 seconds or more). Assess the QT interval against the HR/QTc chart to estimate normal, long, or short QTc.
C) Provide an interpretation.

Clinically Based Critical Thinking: Interpretation

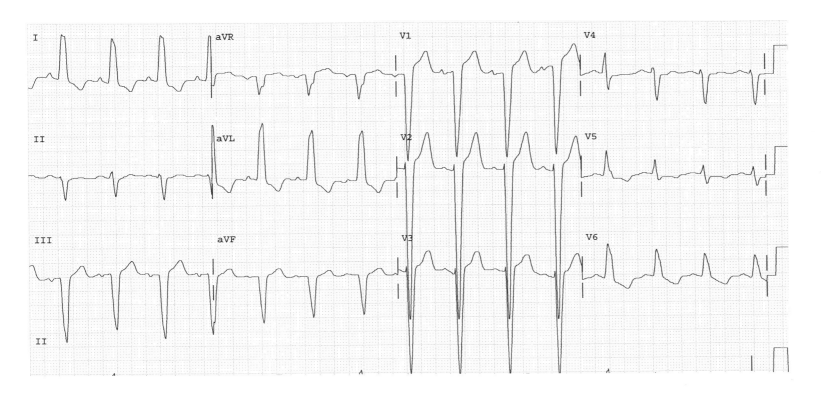

Axis—The Science of Direction

Self-Study Objectives

- Identify and describe the 6 frontal plane leads

- Identify and describe the 6 horizontal plane leads

- Locate leads I, II, III, AVL, AVR, and AVF on the frontal plane diagram

- Locate leads V1, V2, V3, V4, V5, and V6 on the horizontal plane diagram

- Memorize the 3 leads that define:
  a) rightward or leftward
  b) up or down
  c) anterior or posterior

- Distinguish whether a P wave, QRS complex, or T wave is pointing:
  a) rightward or leftward
  b) up or down
  c) anterior or posterior

- Describe the normal P wave direction

- Describe the significance of the P wave direction in determining whether the EKG was taken correctly or the arm leads were mistakenly reversed

- Identify and describe dextrocardia, junctional rhythm, and normal P wave directions.

The heart is a continuously active muscle that pumps blood. Think about that the next time you get on a treadmill, and the next time you think about eating a bacon cheddar cheeseburger. It must also produce electrical and mechanical energy on a continuous basis. Both forms of energy come from specialized cardiac muscle fibers. These fibers provide electrical signals and mechanical energy that physically pumps the blood. Although the EKG does not show that mechanical energy, it can be used to measure a variety of electrical events. Each of these occurs in a normal sequence, in a normal direction, and with a normal magnitude. If we could see this force with our eyes, it could look something like this. The atrial systole (Figure 6.1) would show a small force in the direction of the normal depolarization wave, down and to the patient's left. The ventricular systole (Figure 6.2) would show a similar but much larger force in the same direction. Finally, the ventricles would reset or repolarize (Figure 6.3) with a force and direction that proceeds down and to the patient's left.

Beginning Simply: If Only We Could See Electricity

Of course, we cannot see electricity inside the body with our eyes, but other sensors, called electrocardiographic leads, can see electricity. An EKG has 12 leads, with 6 in the frontal plane, or view, and 6 in the horizontal, or top

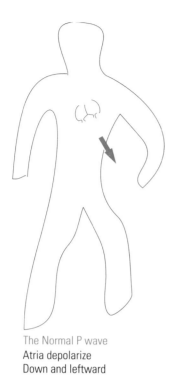

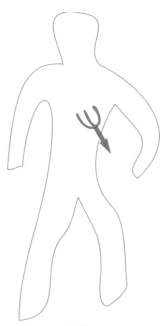

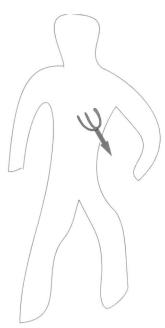

The Normal P wave
Atria depolarize
Down and leftward

FIGURE 6.1

The Normal QRS
Ventricles depolarize
Down and leftward

FIGURE 6.2

The Normal T Wave
Ventricles repolarize
Down and leftward

FIGURE 6.3

down, view. Because these sensors are so primitive, they can sense in one dimension only. Therefore, it is necessary to combine the partial information from each lead with the information from the other leads on the EKG for a complete three-dimensional picture of the electrical forces to emerge. By learning how to combine the "visual" information provided by each of the 12 primitive leads, we can actually reconstruct the direction and force that our eyes would see if we could see electrical events! This EKG in Figure 6.4 has 12 leads or sensors, each of which measures electricity from a different angle or viewpoint. We need to examine all 12 leads above to "see" the electrical force as in Figure 6.5! If you learn to calculate direction, you will be able to "see" the EKG (Figure 6.4) as it looks in Figure 6.5.

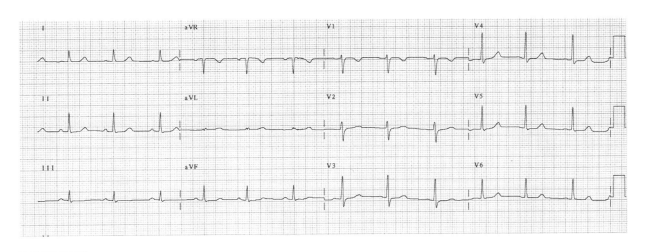

FIGURE 6.4

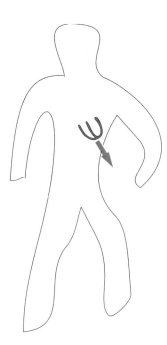

FIGURE 6.5

The 12 Separate EKG Leads
Equal One Arrow Visually

When a force is abnormal in size or direction, it may indicate that the specific part of the heart producing the force is abnormal. Therefore, learning the normal electrical direction of forces in the heart provides a simple and scientific way of understanding and interpreting an EKG. We will learn to measure the electrical direction for the P wave, the QRS complex, and the T wave, as well as for other forces throughout the book. The remainder of this chapter teaches one method for determining the direction of the electrical force for any of these waves, or complexes, on the EKG. By drawing out the electrical forces on paper, we can "see" the electrical force and learn simple concepts to help determine what is normal and what is abnormal. These 12 leads (as in Figure 6.6) usually each have a P wave, a QRS, and a T wave. Taken together, they allow us to "see" the actual electrical forces as though they were externally visible to our eyes. Learn to put the 12 leads into one picture. That is the secret of understanding an EKG!

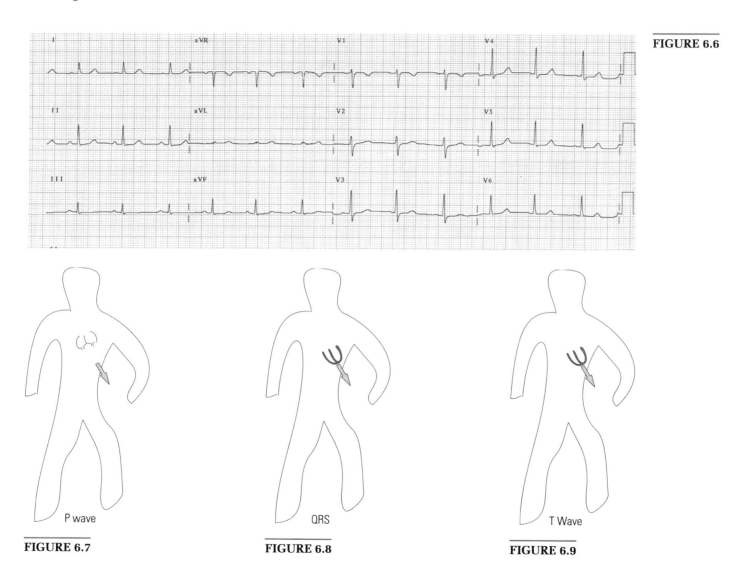

FIGURE 6.6

FIGURE 6.7

FIGURE 6.8

FIGURE 6.9

Begin to Visualize: Draw the Direction Diagram (Memorize!)

When measuring the axis or direction of any force in the frontal plane, begin by drawing and labeling the leads as shown in this representation of a frontal view of the heart. Continue the line segments through the center to the other side of the circle. This results in the second diagram. We now have the six frontal plane sensors arranged in a circle. They will allow us to calculate and then visualize direction as up or down and right or left, within 15 degrees.

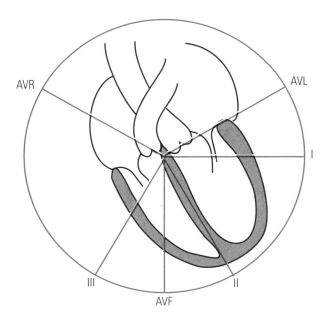

FIGURE 6.10

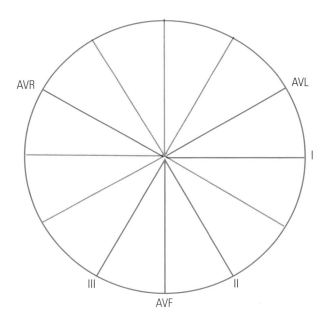

FIGURE 6.11

Add Degrees to the Frontal Plane Direction Diagram

To provide an easy and understandable way to describe direction, label each of the leads in degrees. Lead I is the starting point at 0°. **Continuing counter-clockwise is considered negative, but rotation clockwise from zero is considered positive.** By combining the information from each of these leads (I, II, III, AVR, AVL, AVF), the direction of any electrical force can be converted to a visual image. **To clarify what the diagram represents, try imagining the heart superimposed on top of it. This is actually a way of clearly visualizing the direction of the force moving through the heart.**

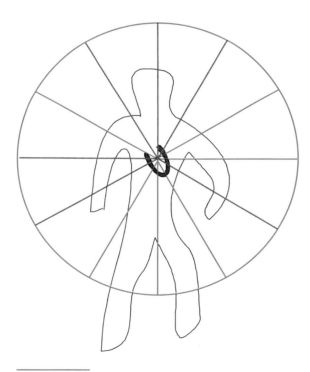

FIGURE 6.12

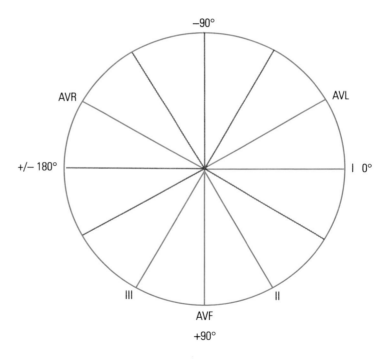

FIGURE 6.13

Diagram Leads as One-Dimensional Sensors or Observers

Place lead I on our diagram. This primitive sensor sees only in one dimension and looks at the view from the patient's left side. It can "sense" whether or not an electrical force is present, tell us if that force is large or small, and also give us a single piece of information on direction. That is, whether the electrical force is going to the patient's left or right side. Each diagram lead senses the patient's P wave, QRS, and T wave. In this example (Figure 6.14), the P wave is upward in lead I. Therefore the atrial force is pointing toward the sensor, and to the patient's left side. The QRS and T wave are normally pointing the same way as the P wave—in this example, to the patient's left. Because this P wave in lead I is mostly upward or positive, we can "see" the P wave as pointing toward the patient's left side. Mathematically, it would be somewhere between −90° and +90°. Visually, we can "see" the P wave as pointing to the patient's left! And, since the QRS and T wave are both positive, we can visualize them as pointing to the patient's left as well.

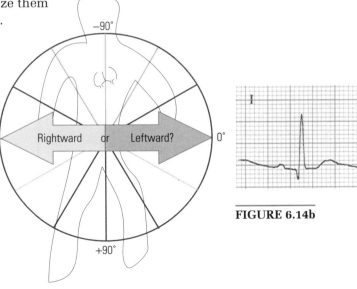

FIGURE 6.14b

FIGURE 6.14a

The Frontal Plane Leads:
Visualizing Right from Left—Lead I

Remember that each lead is so primitive that it can "see" in only one dimension and can sense only if the electrical force is coming toward it or going away from it. **Using this method, examine the P wave in lead I first. Your perspective is that of someone viewing the cardiac events from this location. The sensor at lead I is perfectly placed to provide one critical piece of information, namely whether the electrical force is pointing left or right.** If the P wave (or any wave for that matter) is upright or positive, then the observer visualizes that force as pointing toward the patient's left side. **If the lead I sensor is negative or downward, the observer visualizes the force as pointing toward the patient's right side.** This concept of "positive = toward" and "negative = away" relative to any of the EKG leads is fundamental to visualizing direction.

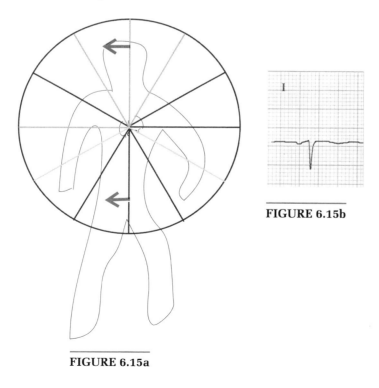

FIGURE 6.15b

FIGURE 6.15a

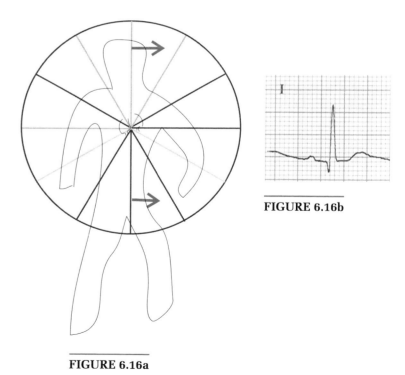

FIGURE 6.16b

FIGURE 6.16a

The Frontal Plane Leads: Visualizing Up and Down—Lead AVF

Once again, remember that each of the 12 EKG leads is so primitive it can "see" only one in dimension and can sense only if an electrical force is coming toward it or going away from it. Lead I has already let the observer visualize whether the force is pointing right or left. Lead AVF is the sensor below the patient's feet and provides the perspective of someone viewing the cardiac events from below. The sensor at lead AVF is perfectly placed to provide another critical piece of information, namely whether the electrical force is pointing up or down. If the P wave (or any wave for that matter) is upright or positive, then the observer visualizes that force as pointing toward the patient's feet, which is where AVF is placed. If the lead AVF sensor is negative or downward, then the observer visualizes the force as pointing toward the patient's head. Be careful with AVF! If *lead AVF is "up," then visualize the* force as "downward!"

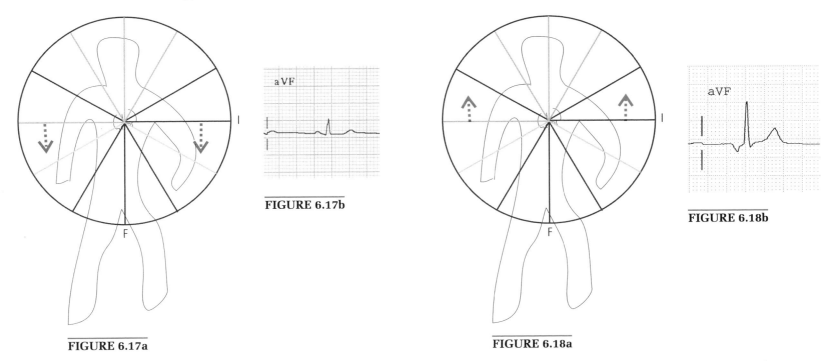

FIGURE 6.17b

FIGURE 6.18b

FIGURE 6.17a

FIGURE 6.18a

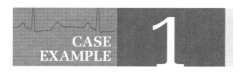

How Leads Determine Direction

How Lead I Separates Left from Right

For this example, let's visualize ventricular electrical systole, which is represented by the QRS. To determine and visualize whether the QRS is pointing, right or left, as well as up or down, first examine lead I. Because lead I is positive, the QRS is visualized as pointing toward the patient's left. This is not yet a complete description or picture.

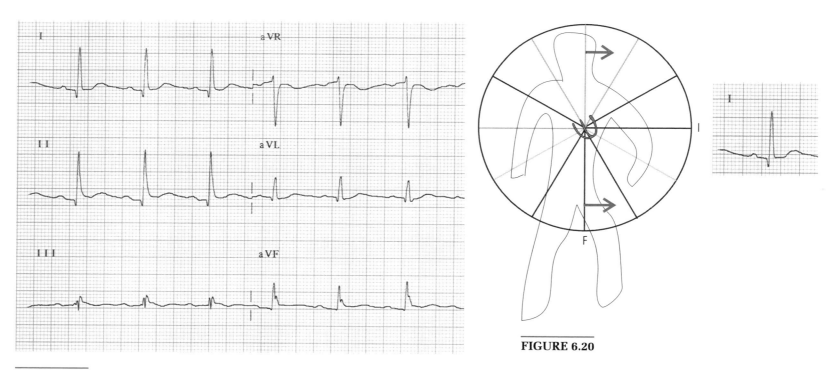

FIGURE 6.20

FIGURE 6.19

How Lead AVF Tells Up from Down (CAREFUL!)

Because the QRS in Lead I was positive, the QRS was visualized as pointing to the patient's left side. To help complete the visualization, the observer needs to next determine whether the QRS force is toward the patient's head or feet as well. The sensor that can distinguish up from down is called lead AVF. As lead AVF is positive, the observer visualizes the QRS as pointing toward the patient's feet, that is, inferiorly. This can seem totally counterintuitive, so go over this page very carefully!

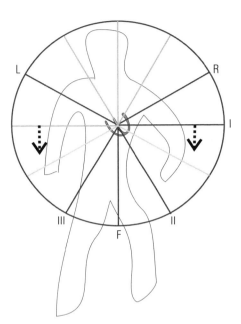

FIGURE 6.22a

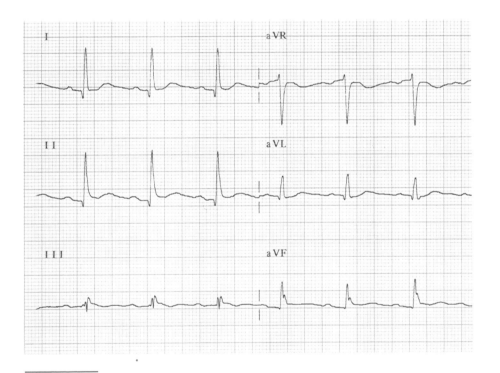

FIGURE 6.21

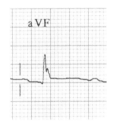

FIGURE 6.22b

How Combining Leads I and AVF Determines a Quadrant

Although the information from leads I and AVF was drawn on separate diagrams for purposes of illustration, drawing them on one diagram helps construct a more complete visualizion. Looking at leads I and AVF together will narrow the direction to one of the four quadrants. In this example, the QRS axis lies below line I and to the left of line AVF, or in the lower left quadrant. (Mathematically, the axis is greater than 0° and less than positive 90°.) Remember that (a) any electrical event (P wave, QRS, T wave, anything else!) that is above the baseline in lead I can be visualized as pointing to the patient's left, and (b) any electrical event that is above the baseline in lead AVF is pointing toward the patient's feet, that is, inferiorly (See Figure 6.63).

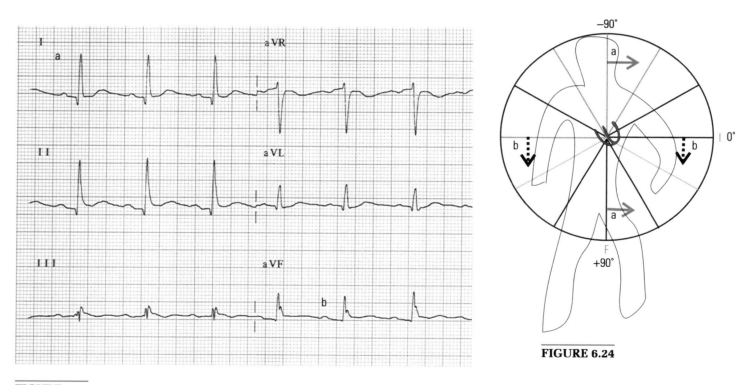

FIGURE 6.23

FIGURE 6.24

Visualizing More Precisely Within a Quadrant

Using lead I and lead AVF will narrow down any force to one of the four quadrants on the diagram. In this example, because leads I and AVF are positive, the observer can visualize the QRS and ventricular depolarization as grossly pointing down and to the patient's left. For greater accuracy, the axis can be narrowed down further to a multiple of 15°, as shown in Figure 6.25. To calculate the axis to multiples of 15°, additional information is needed from the other four one-dimensional sensors: leads II, III, AVR, and AVL. With the information from these leads, the observer can narrow the visualization down to one of the arrows.

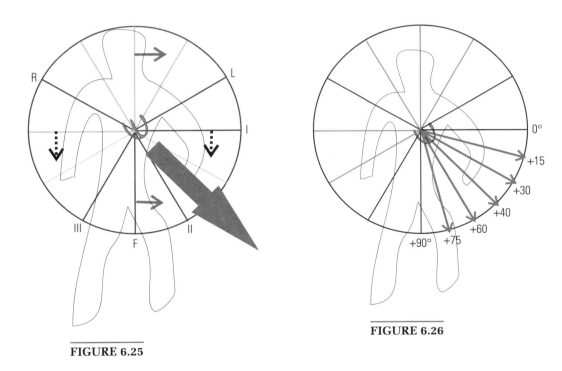

FIGURE 6.25

FIGURE 6.26

Narrowing Down the Direction with Lead III

To determine the exact direction inside a quadrant, the observer can look at a lead OUTSIDE the quadrant. In this example, leads III, AVR, and AVL lie outside the lower left quadrant. Again, each of the 12 EKG leads is so primitive it can "see" only in one dimension and can sense only if an electrical force is coming toward it or going away from it. Lead III gives the observer the perspective from the patient's lower right side.

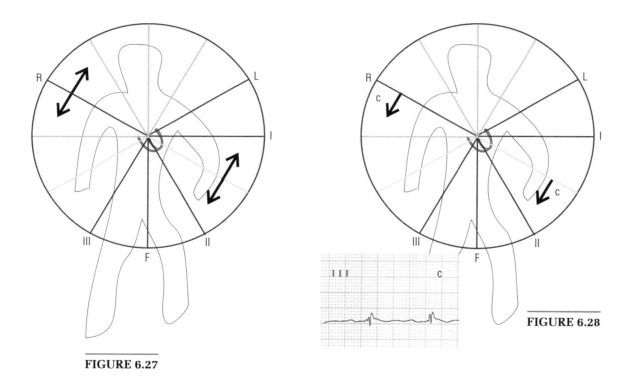

FIGURE 6.27

FIGURE 6.28

Combining the Information—Leads I, AVF, and III

Combine the directional information from the three leads (I, AVF, and III) into one diagram.

- **a.** Lead I is positive
- **b.** Lead AVF is positive
- **c.** Lead III is positive

Using a, b, and c, from above, the visualized direction is greater than +30 and less than +90 degrees. Since we are using multiples of 15, the axis must be +45, +60, or +75 degrees.

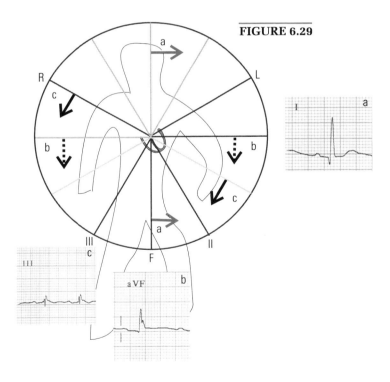

FIGURE 6.29

Finalizing the Direction with Lead AVL

To narrow down the exact direction inside a quadrant, the oberver can again look at a lead OUTSIDE the quadrant. In this example, AVR and AVL lie outside the lower left quadrant. Again, each of the 12 EKG leads is so primitive it can "see" only one in dimension and can sense only if an electrical force is coming toward it or going away from it. Lead AVL offers the observer the perspective from the patient's left shoulder.

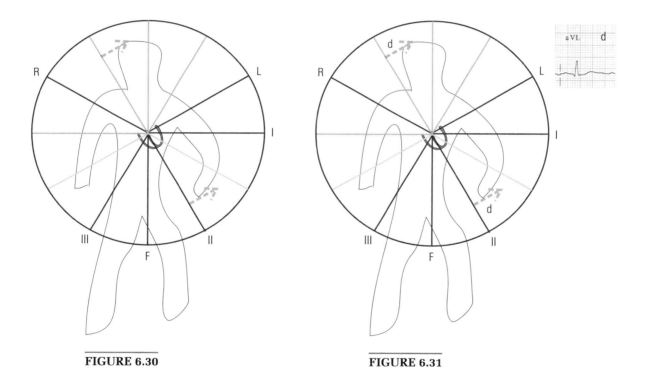

FIGURE 6.30   **FIGURE 6.31**

Summary and Conclusion—Step by Step

We have determined that:

a)	Lead I is positive	which told us the QRS direction is to the patient's left side
b)	Lead AVF is positive	which told us the QRS direction is to the patient's feet
c)	Lead III is positive	which told us the QRS direction was >30 degrees
d)	Lead AVL is positive	which told us the QRS direction was <60 degrees, and so QED +45!

And all that information is equivalent to just saying the QRS direction is +45!

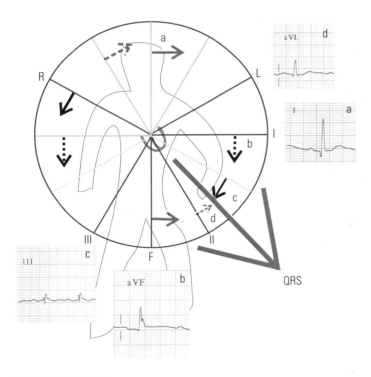

FIGURE 6.32a–d

CASE EXAMPLE 2 Another Example of Normal

Let the observer construct another example of normal in which Lead III is isoelectric, that is, neither obviously positive or negative.

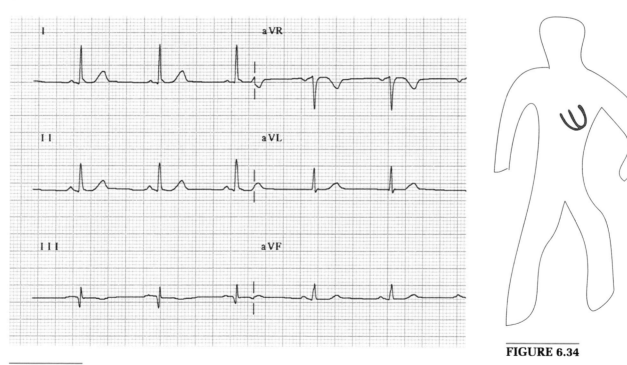

FIGURE 6.33

FIGURE 6.34

Always Begin with Lead I and Lead AVF

In this example, the QRS in Lead I is positive, and so points to the patient's left side. The QRS is positive in Lead AVF (careful!). It so points toward the lead and, therefore, downward towards the patient's feet (see Figure 6.63).

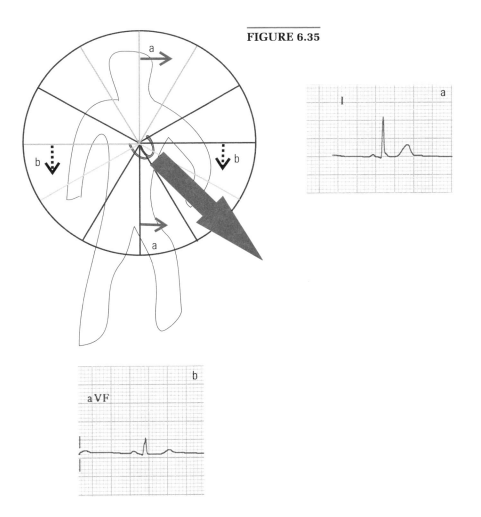

FIGURE 6.35

How to Handle an Isoelectric Lead

In this example, the positive QRS in lead I and positive QRS in lead AVF lets the observer visualize the direction as down and to the patient's left side. (Mathematically, QRS direction is expressed as somewhere between 0° and 90°.) To narrow down the direction more precisely, look at another lead outside the lower left quadrant. Lead III or lead AVL would help. For this example, arbitrarily select Lead III to examine first. The observer sees that the QRS in lead III is neither obviously positive or negative. This is called an isoelectric lead. When a lead is isoelectric, it provides a helpful and specific clue, because the true direction must be perpendicular to this lead.

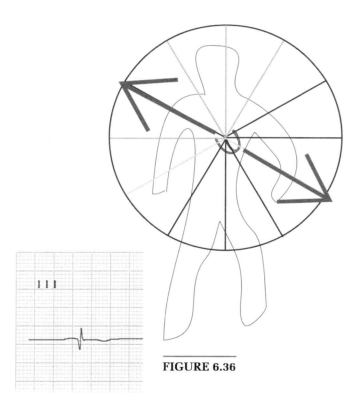

FIGURE 6.36

Summary and Conclusion—Step by Step

We have determined that

a) Lead I is positive — which told us the QRS direction is to the patient's left side

b) Lead AVF is positive — which told us the QRS direction is to the patient's feet

c) Lead III is isoelectric — which told us the QRS direction was either −150° or +30°

And all that information is equivalent to just saying the QRS direction is +30! This is a normal QRS direction.

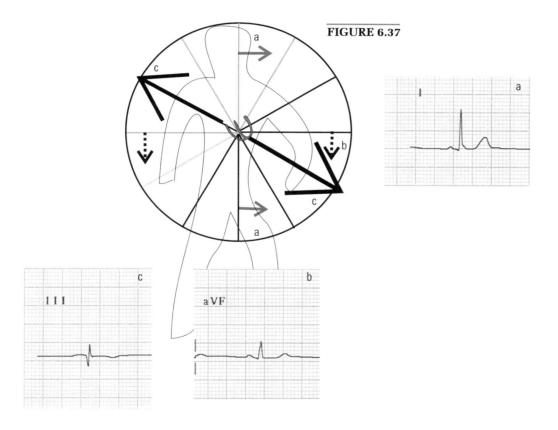

FIGURE 6.37

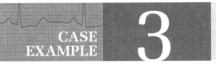

Abnormal QRS Direction in the Frontal Plane

CASE EXAMPLE 3

Begin at the beginning with Lead I. In this example, Lead I is positive, so the QRS direction is to the patient's left side. Mathematically, the QRS is somewhere between −90° and +90°.

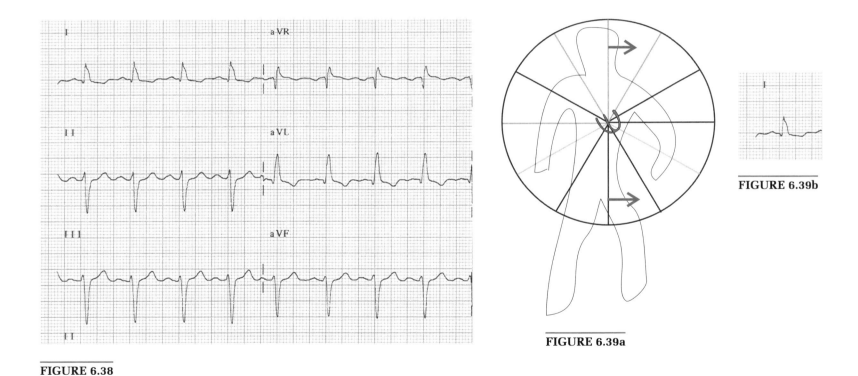

FIGURE 6.38

FIGURE 6.39a

FIGURE 6.39b

Abnormal QRS Direction in the Frontal Plane

Lead AVF is negative. This means the QRS direction is away from Lead AVF or upward. (Always be very careful thinking about lead AVF. It is very easy to make a careless mistake with this lead!) **It is not normal for the QRS direction to be upward, so the oberver needs to determine the direction more precisely. Although diagnostic possibilities include inferior infarction and left anterior hemiblock, do not worry about the diagnosis yet. These will be covered in depth in later chapters. Focus on learning to differentiate up from down and left from right (Figure 6.63)!**

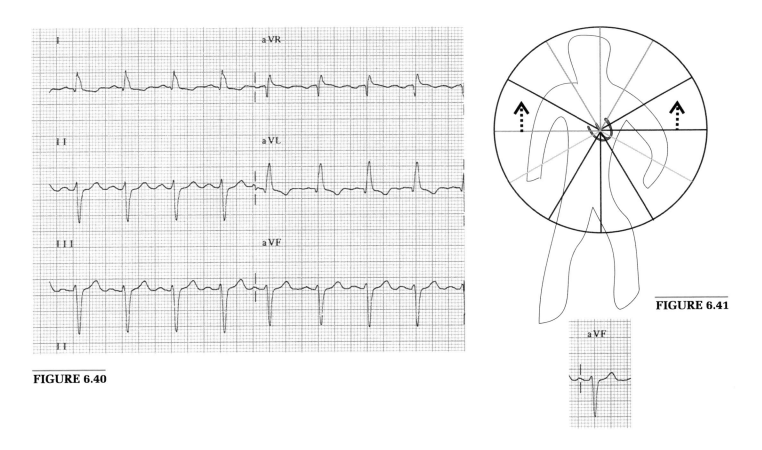

FIGURE 6.40

FIGURE 6.41

Abnormal QRS Direction in the Frontal Plane

Combining the information from leads I and AVF, as was done in the previous examples, visualize the QRS direction to be leftward and upward.

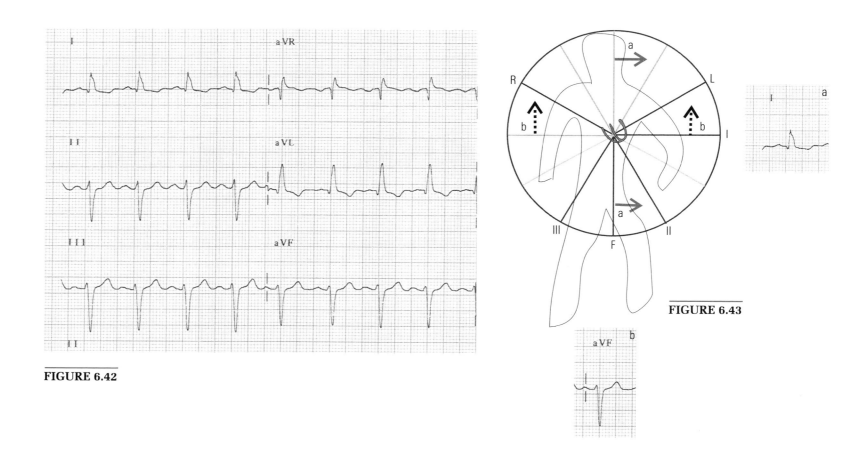

FIGURE 6.42

FIGURE 6.43

Abnormal QRS Direction in the Frontal Plane

The positive QRS in lead I and negative QRS in lead AVF let the observer visualize the direction to the patient's left side and upward. **Mathematically, the QRS direction is somewhere between 0° and −90°. To narrow down the direction more precisely, look at another lead outside the left upward quadrant. Lead II or lead AVR would help. For this example, arbitrarily examine Lead II. The QRS in Lead II is negative.** Because Lead II records the QRS as negative, the QRS is going away from lead II.

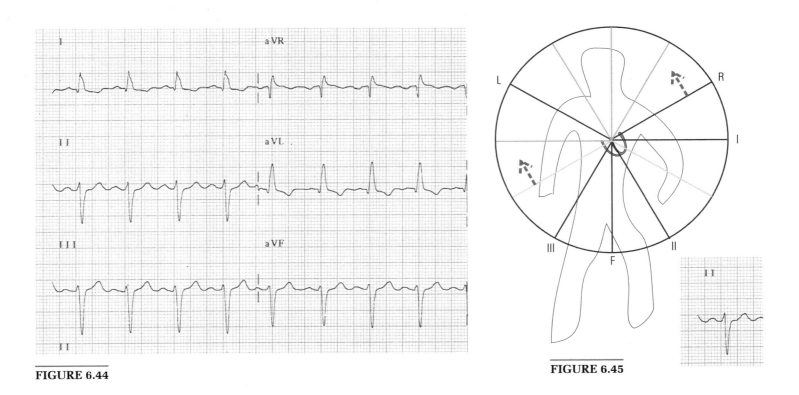

FIGURE 6.44

FIGURE 6.45

Abnormal QRS Direction in the Frontal Plane

Now combine the information from Lead II with the information from leads I and AVF onto one diagram. Using the information from lead I (a), the QRS direction is to the patient's left side. Using the information from lead AVF (b), the QRS direction is upward, superiorly, to the patient's head. (Mathematically, the direction is visualized as between 0 and −90°.) Lead II is negative, thus the observer can visualize the QRS as also pointing away from lead II. Now the direction is visualized as somewhere between −30° and −90°. The direction can be determined even more precisely by looking at another lead outside the upper left quadrant, namely lead AVR.

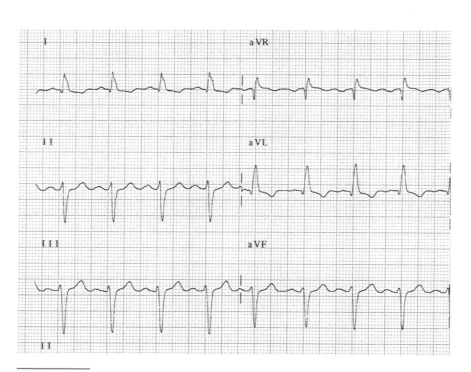

FIGURE 6.46

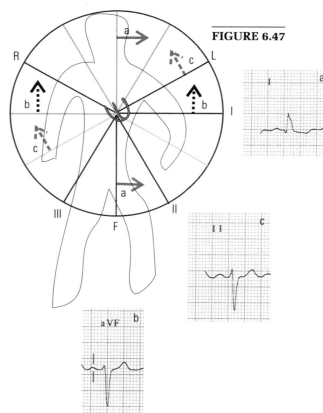

FIGURE 6.47

Abnormal QRS Direction in the Frontal Plane

To improve visualization, add information from another lead outside the upper left quadrant, namely lead AVR. In this example, lead AVR is slightly more positive than negative. Therefore the QRS direction is headed toward lead AVR.

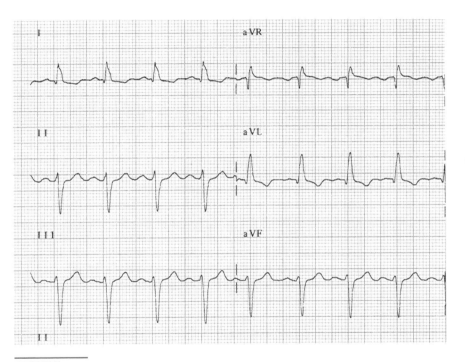

FIGURE 6.48

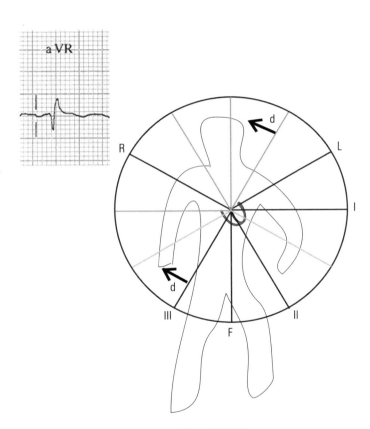

FIGURE 6.49

Summary and Conclusion—Step by Step

We have determined that

a) Lead I is positive   which told us the QRS direction is leftward

b) Lead AVF is negative   which told us the QRS direction is upward or superiorly

c) Lead II is negative   which told us the QRS direction was < −30 degrees

d) Lead AVR is positive   which told us the QRS direction was < −60 degrees, and so must be −75°!

And all that information is exactly equivalent to just saying the QRS direction is −75°! This QRS direction is abnormal.

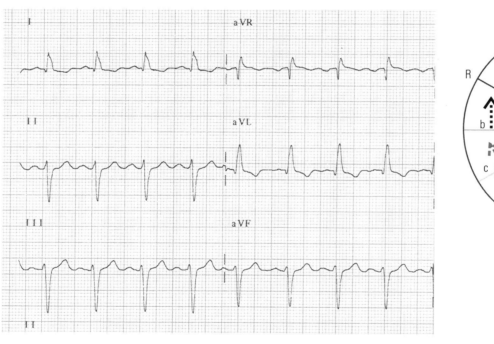

FIGURE 6.50

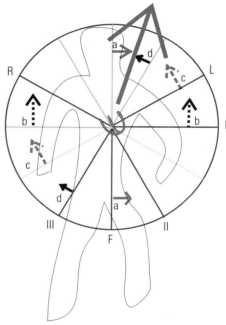

FIGURE 6.51

The View from the Top:
The Horizontal Plane

Space has three dimensions. So do all living things. So far, we visualized the heart in two dimensions: (1) up and down and (2) left and right. The third dimension, the horizontal plane, looks at the body and the heart from above. It visualizes right and left, but instead of up and down, it shows if the electrical force is moving frontward (anterior) or backward (posterior).

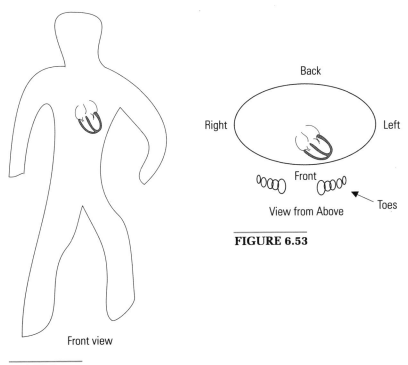

Front view

FIGURE 6.52

Back

Right   Left

Front

View from Above   Toes

FIGURE 6.53

Draw the Horizontal Plane Diagram

Lead V2 is directly anterior. Lead V6 is at the patient's left.

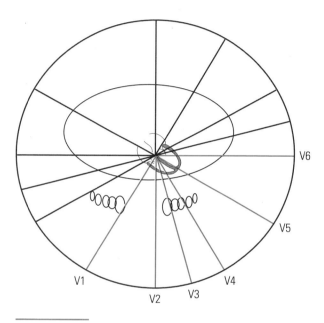

FIGURE 6.54

Horizontal Plane Diagram:
Labeling the Degree Increments

Lead V6 is arbitrarily considered to be 0°. Counterclockwise from V6 is negative. Clockwise from V6 is positive.

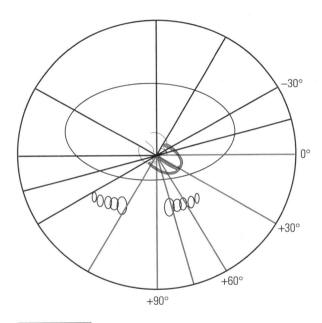

−30°

0°

+30°

+60°

+90°

FIGURE 6.55

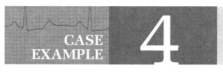

Using the Frontal Plane and the Horizontal Plane

Examine this EKG, and visualize the QRS direction in 3 dimensions.

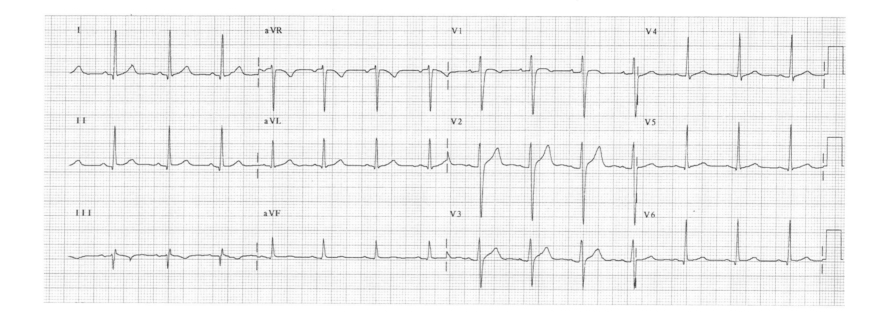

The Frontal Plane Step by Step

We have determined that

a) Lead I is positive   which told us the QRS direction is leftward

b) Lead AVF is positive   which told us the QRS direction is downward or inferiorly

c) Lead III is negative   which told us the QRS direction was <+30° , and so the direction is +15°

And all that information is exactly equivalent to just saying the QRS direction is +15°! This QRS direction is normal.

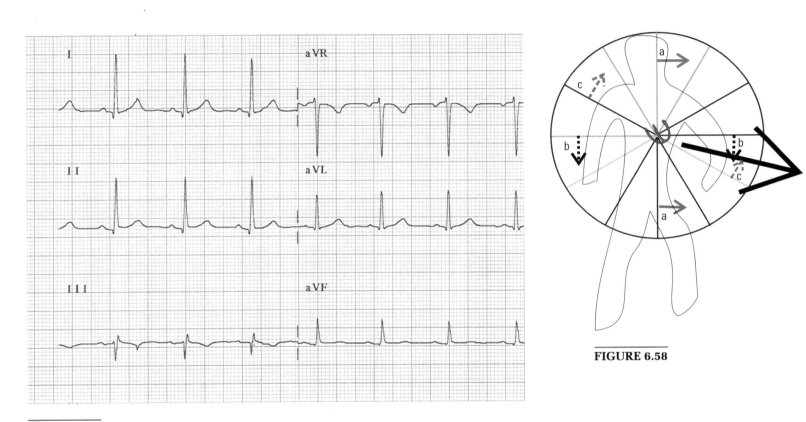

FIGURE 6.58

FIGURE 6.57

Next Assess the Horizontal Leads

Begin with V6. Since the QRS is positive in V6, the direction is toward the patient's left side. The QRS is negative in V2. Therefore we visualize the QRS as pointing toward the patient's back, which is normal.

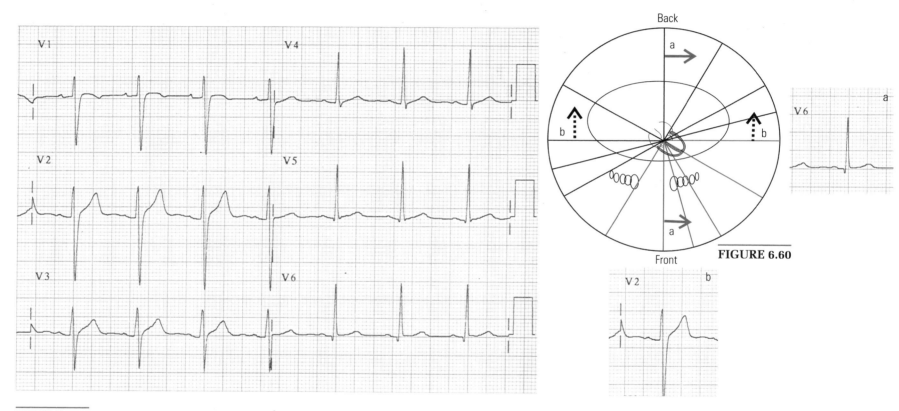

FIGURE 6.59

FIGURE 6.60

3D Summary and Conclusion—Step by Step

We have determined that

a) Lead I is positive — which told us the QRS direction is leftward
b) Lead AVF is positive — which told us the QRS direction is downward or inferior
c) Lead III is negative — which told us the QRS direction was <+30 degrees
d) Lead V2 is negative — which told us the QRS direction was posterior!

And all that information is equivalent to saying the QRS direction is at +15° in the frontal plane and pointing posteriorly in the horizontal plane! This QRS direction is normal. Practice these visualizations thoroughly, and you will find the rest of the book reduces to very simple concepts.

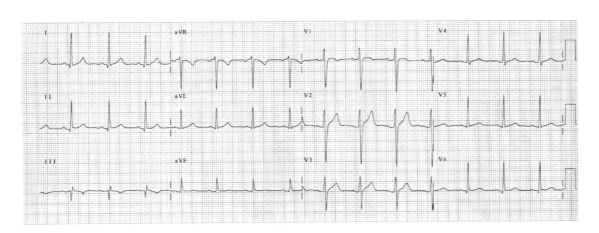

FIGURE 6.61

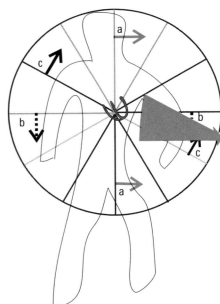

FIGURE 6.62

MEMORIZE THIS!   **The Three Key Leads to Visualization!**

Any P, or QRS, or T wave that is. . . .

upward in Lead I is pointing to the patient's left side,   BUT downward in lead I is pointing to the patient's right side.
upward in Lead AVF is pointing inferiorly (careful!),   BUT downward in lead AVF is pointing superiorly. (careful!)
upward in Lead V2 is pointing anteriorly,   BUT downward in lead V2 is pointing posteriorly.

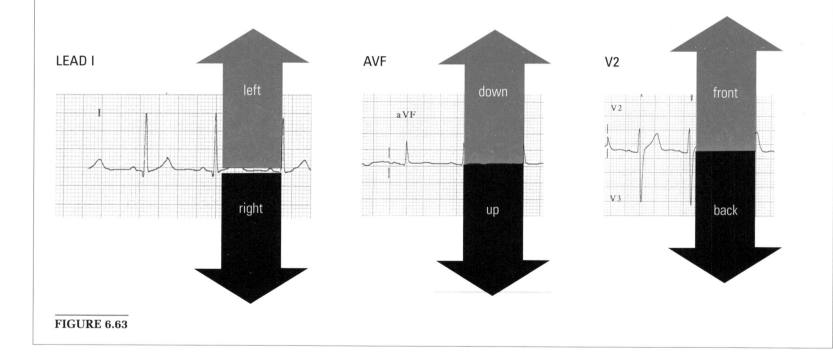

FIGURE 6.63

The P Wave Direction:
Normally Inferiorly and to the Left

Depolarization of the right atrium and left atrium causes an electrical force that appears on the EKG as a P wave. **The P wave has a normal direction based on this normal physiology. The electrical impulse is expected to travel through the atria toward the AV node in a direction (Figure 6.64a) that is downward and to the left. Therefore,** the P wave would typically be positive in lead I (leftward) and positive in lead AVF (inferior) as well.

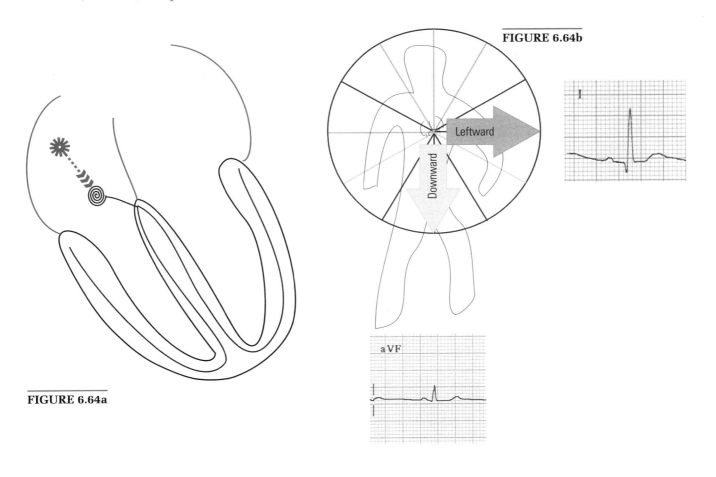

FIGURE 6.64b

FIGURE 6.64a

The P Wave Direction: Arm Lead Misplacement

Always check the P wave direction on every EKG. An upside down P wave in lead I (Figure 6.65 and 6.66b) suggests that the EKG was taken with the arm leads accidentally reversed on the patient's arms. **This results in a right-to-left reversal of direction of what the EKG sees, as is shown in Figure 6.65.** Always check that the P wave direction is as expected to ensure that the EKG was taken correctly!

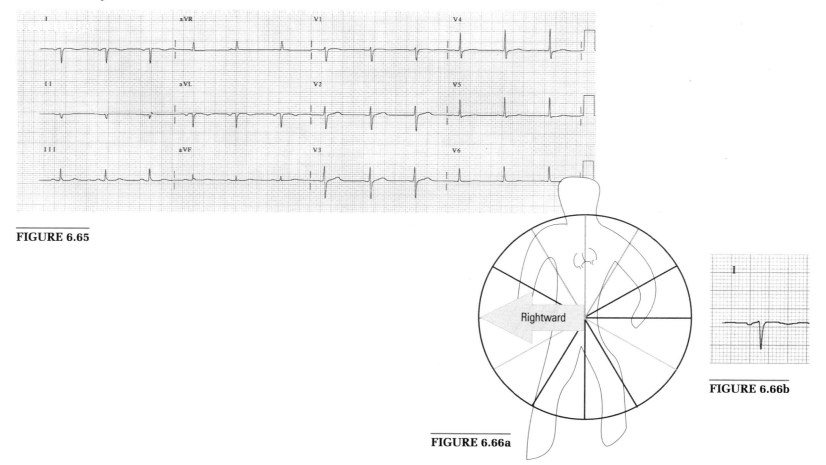

FIGURE 6.65

FIGURE 6.66a

FIGURE 6.66b

The P Wave Direction: Dextrocardia

A P direction that is rightward (positive in lead I) suggests dextrocardia, as well as possible arm lead reversal. **Dextrocardia is a congenital condition in which the contents of the thorax and abdomen are reversed in placement in a mirror image from normal. The difference is seen in the V leads. In arm lead reversal, the V leads appear normal.** In dextrocardia, the V leads are on the opposite side of the chest from the heart. This results in the tell-tale decremental size of the QRS as one moves from lead V1 to lead V6.

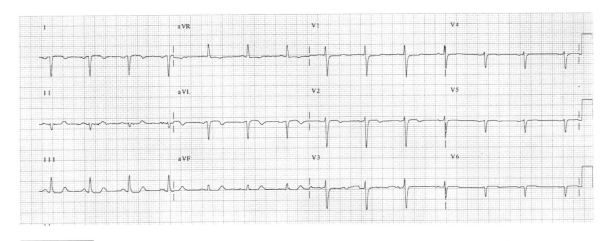

FIGURE 6.67

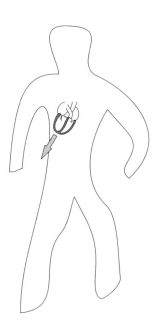

FIGURE 6.68

The P Wave Direction: Junctional Rhythm

Normally, the direction of atrial depolarization is from the sinus node to the AV node, which is from top to bottom. The observer sees this as a P wave direction that points downward and to the patient's left side. In abnormal situations, the junction can start the rhythm and depolarize the atria from the AV node upward. This changes the atrial depolarization and P wave from downward to upward. An upward (relative to the patient) P wave direction (P wave is negative in leads II, III, and AVF) suggests junctional rhythm.

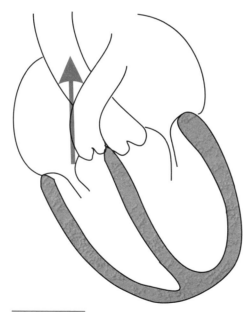

FIGURE 6.69

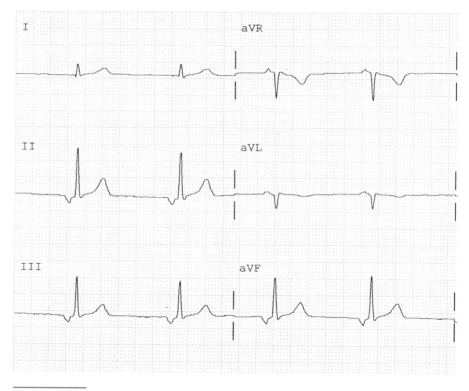

FIGURE 6.70

The P Wave Direction:
Step by Step to Diagnosis

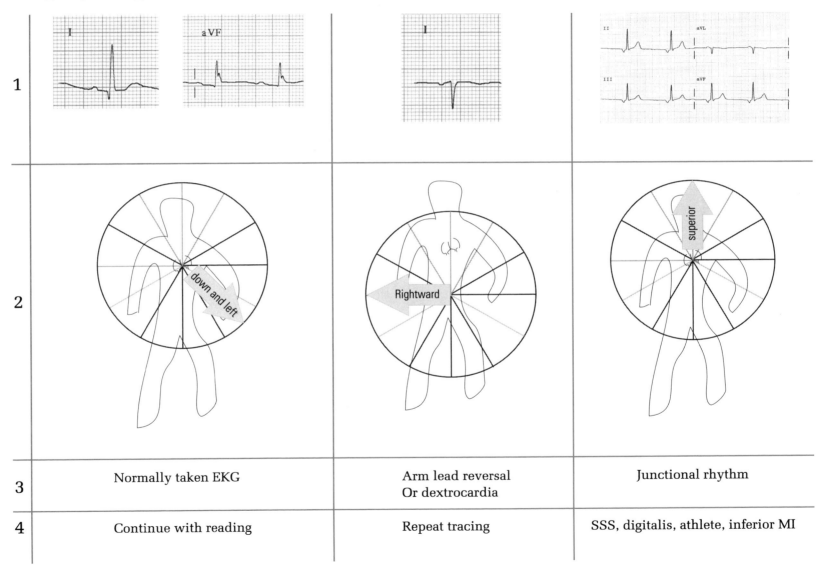

1			
2			
3	Normally taken EKG	Arm lead reversal Or dextrocardia	Junctional rhythm
4	Continue with reading	Repeat tracing	SSS, digitalis, athlete, inferior MI

SAMPLE COMPLETED WORKSHEET

BASIC MEASUREMENTS

Parameter	Measurement	Interpretation
HR	75	Abnormal
Rhythm	Sinus Tach	Abnormal
PR	0.12	Normal
QRS	0.08	Normal
QT	0.36	
QTc	0.40	Normal
P direction	Inferior and leftward	Normal
QRS direction		

Instructions for Chapter 6 Worksheets

A) Complete basic measurements.
B) Describe or calculate the P direction in the frontal plane as inferior or superior, leftward or rightward. Diagnose the P direction as normal if it is inferior and leftward. Diagnose junctional rhythm if the P direction is superior. Diagnose as possible arm lead reversal or dextrocardia if the P wave direction is rightward.
C) Provide an interpretation.

Clinically Based Critical Thinking: Interpretation

Sinus rhythm indicates a balance between the sympathetic and parasympathetic influences on the sinus node. A normal P direction demonstrates that the EKG was taken with the leads correctly placed and can be further interpreted

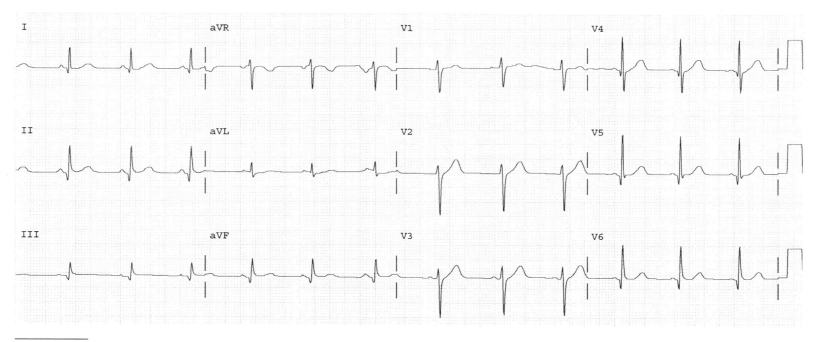

FIGURE 6.72

WORKSHEET 6.1

BASIC MEASUREMENTS		
Parameter	**Measurement**	**Interpretation**
HR		
Rhythm		
PR		
QRS		
QT		
QTc		
P direction		
QRS direction		

Instructions for Chapter 6 Worksheets

A) Complete basic measurements.
B) Describe or calculate the P direction in the frontal plane as inferior or superior, leftward or rightward. Diagnose the P direction as normal if it is inferior and leftward. Diagnose junctional rhythm if the P direction is superior. Diagnose as possible arm lead reversal or dextrocardia if the P wave direction is rightward.
C) Provide an interpretation.

Clinically Based Critical Thinking: Interpretation

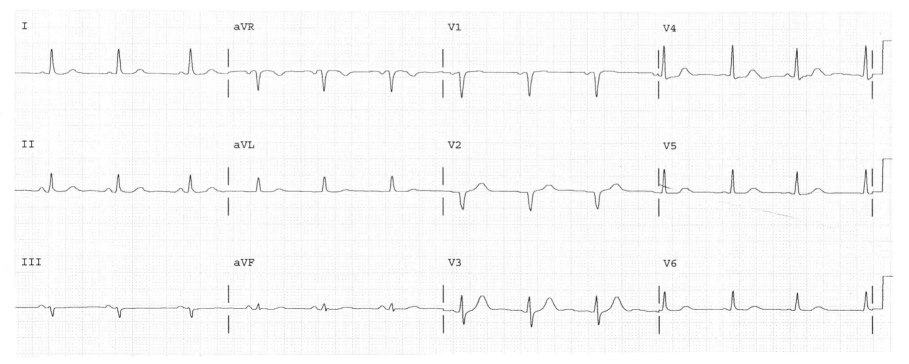

BASIC MEASUREMENTS		
Parameter	**Measurement**	**Interpretation**
HR		
Rhythm		
PR		
QRS		
QT		
QTc		
P direction		
QRS direction		

Instructions for Chapter 6 Worksheets

A) Complete basic measurements.
B) Describe or calculate the P direction in the frontal plane as inferior or superior, leftward or rightward. Diagnose the P direction as normal if it is inferior and leftward. Diagnose junctional rhythm if the P direction is superior. Diagnose as possible arm lead reversal or dextrocardia if the P wave direction is rightward.
C) Provide an interpretation.

Clinically Based Critical Thinking: Interpretation

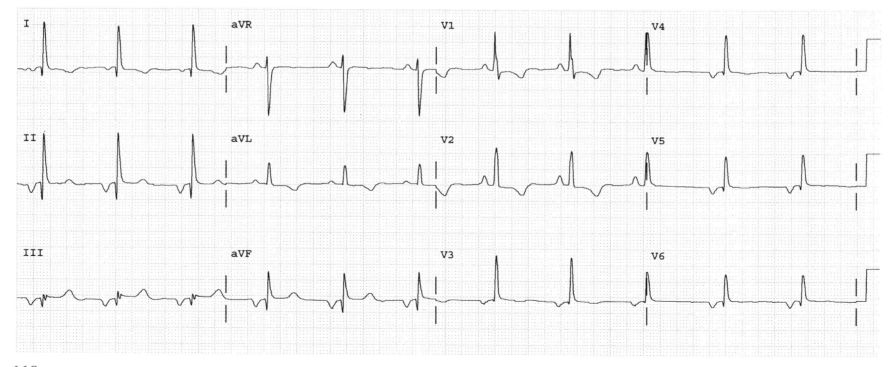

WORKSHEET 6.3

BASIC MEASUREMENTS

Parameter	Measurement	Interpretation
HR		
Rhythm		
PR		
QRS		
QT		
QTc		
P direction		
QRS direction		

Instructions for Chapter 6 Worksheets

A) Complete basic measurements.
B) Describe or calculate the P direction in the frontal plane as inferior or superior, leftward or rightward. Diagnose the P direction as normal if it is inferior and leftward. Diagnose junctional rhythm if the P direction is superior. Diagnose as possible arm lead reversal or dextrocardia if the P wave direction is rightward.
C) Provide an interpretation.

Clinically Based Critical Thinking: Interpretation

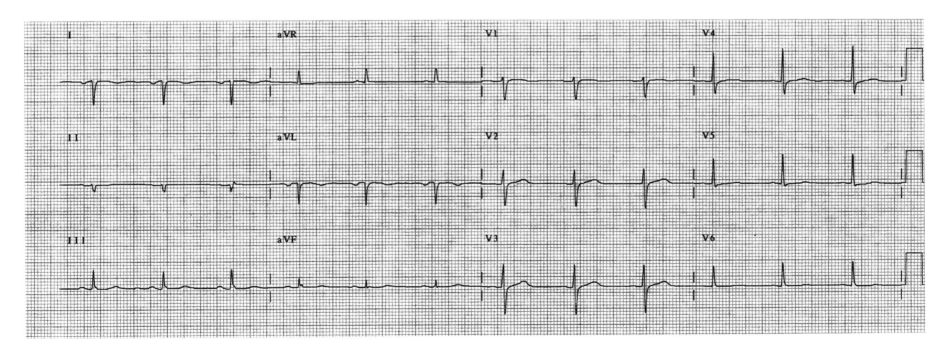

WORKSHEET II.1

BASIC MEASUREMENTS

Parameter	Measurement	Interpretation
HR		
Rhythm		
PR		
QRS		
QT		
QTc		
P direction		
QRS direction		

Clinically Based Critical Thinking: Interpretation

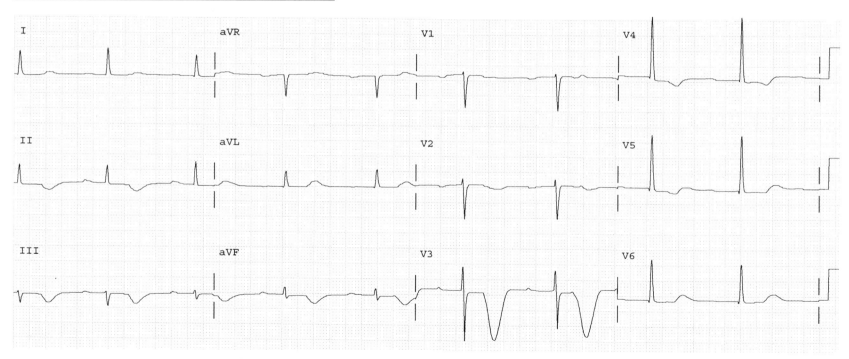

BASIC MEASUREMENTS		
Parameter	Measurement	Interpretation
HR		
Rhythm		
PR		
QRS		
QT		
QTc		
P direction		
QRS direction		

Clinically Based Critical Thinking: Interpretation

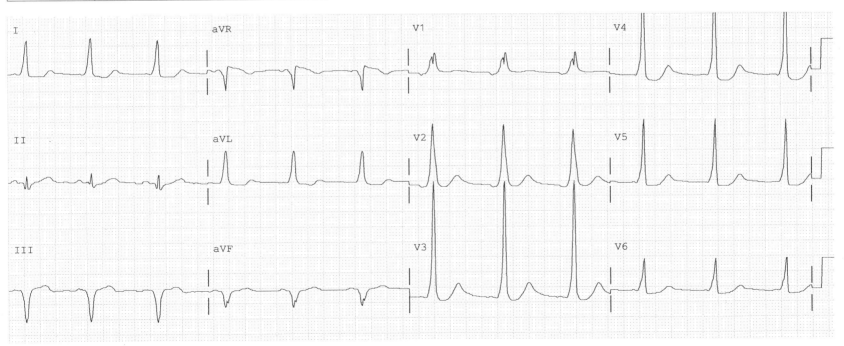

BASIC MEASUREMENTS		
Parameter	Measurement	Interpretation
HR		
Rhythm		
PR		
QRS		
QT		
QTc		
P direction		
QRS direction		

Clinically Based Critical Thinking: Interpretation

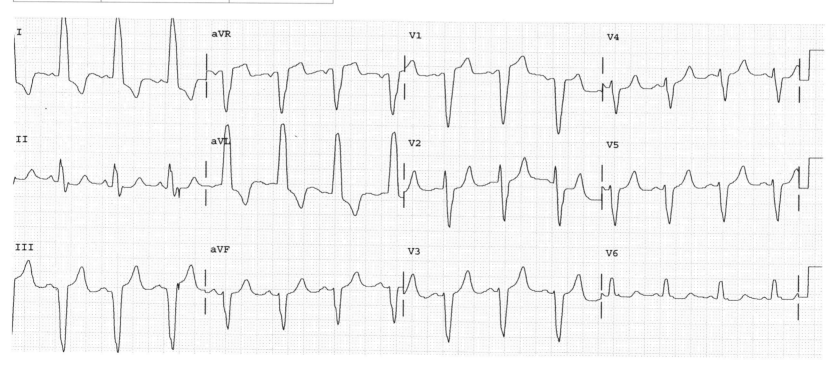

WORKSHEET II.4

BASIC MEASUREMENTS		
Parameter	Measurement	Interpretation
HR		
Rhythm		
PR		
QRS		
QT		
QTc		
P direction		
QRS direction		

Clinically Based Critical Thinking: Interpretation

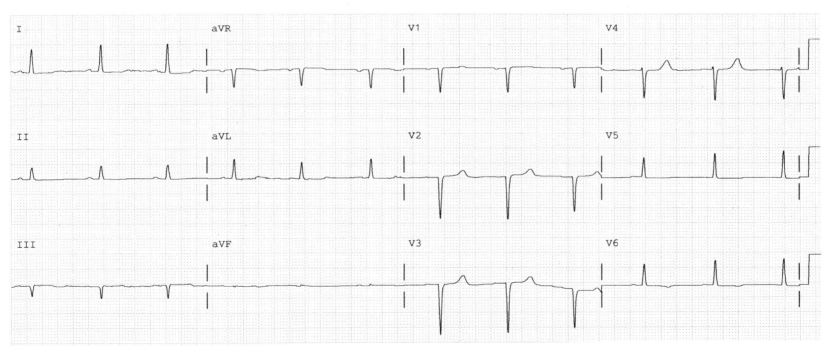

WORKSHEET II.5

BASIC MEASUREMENTS		
Parameter	Measurement	Interpretation
HR		
Rhythm		
PR		
QRS		
QT		
QTc		
P direction		
QRS direction		

Clinically Based Critical Thinking: Interpretation

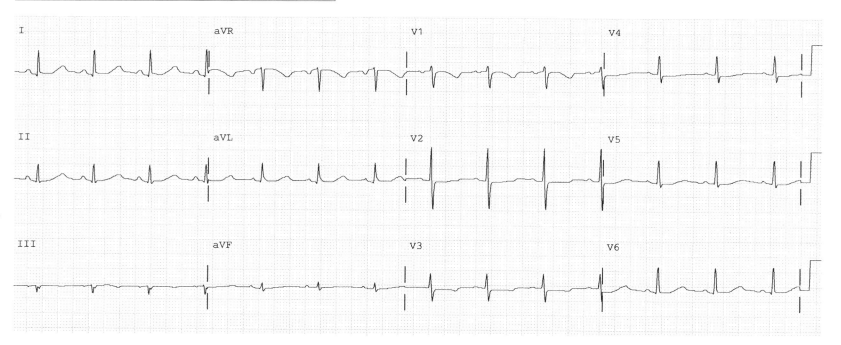

Common Clinical Arrhythmias

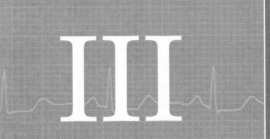

III

Atrial Arrhythmias

Sinus Rhythm

Sinus rhythm is a regular rhythm, with a rate of 60 to 100 beats per minute (bpm). The interval between P waves is constant. A QRS follows each P wave at a constant interval. The heart rate in Figure 7.1 is 68 bpm.

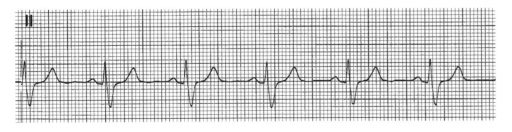

FIGURE 7.1

Sinus Tachycardia

Sinus tachycardia is a regular rhythm, with a rate greater than 100 bpm. **The maximum rate of sinus tachycardia depends on a person's age and can be estimated by the formula** (Max HR = 220 − person's age). **A QRS follows each P wave at a constant interval. The heart rate in Figure 7.2 is 107 bpm.** Sinus tachycardia always has an underlying cause. **The pathophysiology is most commonly sympathetic over activity, but it can be parasympathetic block.**

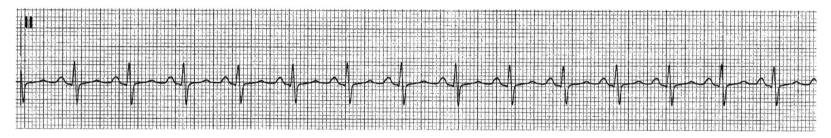

FIGURE 7.2

Sinus Arrhythmia

Sinus arrhythmia is a rhythm characterized by a gradually increasing, then decreasing heart rate, over a period of seconds. **The variation between the maximum (88 bpm) and minimum (75 bpm) heart rates in Figure 7.3 is greater than 10%. A QRS follows each P wave. When marked, it can be a sign of further conduction disease called** sick sinus syndrome.

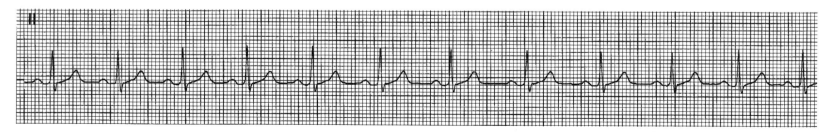

FIGURE 7.3

Sinus Bradycardia

Sinus bradycardia (SB) is a regular rhythm, with a rate of less than 60 bpm. A QRS follows each P wave at a constant interval, and the interval between P waves is constant. The heart rate in Figure 7.4 goes down to 45 bpm. Sinus bradycardia is the result of decreased sympathetic or increased para-sympathetic activity. The class of medications called beta blockers commonly cause sinus bradycardia.

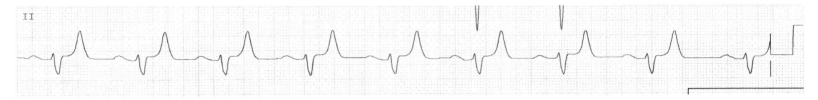

FIGURE 7.4

Atrial Tachycardia

Atrial tachycardia (AT) or supraventricular tachycardia (SVT) is a regular rhythm at a rate of 160 to 260. A P wave, if present (P′), appears differently from the normal P wave (P). The heart rate in Figure 7.5 increases from 91 to more than 160 bpm. Atrial tachycardia is usually associated with increased sympathetic activity. It can be seen in normal and abnormal hearts.

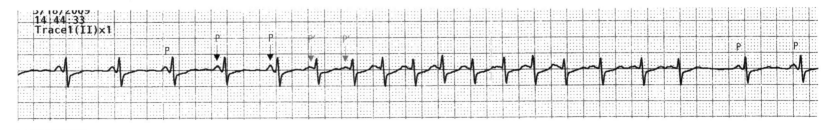

FIGURE 7.5

Atrial Flutter

Atrial flutter is a regular atrial rhythm characterized by atrial flutter waves. Lead II frequently demonstrates the classic sawtooth appearance of the flutter waves, some of which are hidden in the ST segment. Atrial flutter usually is a regular rhythm at a rate of 240 to 340 with flutter waves, but not every flutter wave produces a QRS. The number of flutter waves to QRS complex in Figure 7.6 is described as flutter with varying 3 to 1 and 2 to 1 conduction. The atrial rate (230) and ventricular rate (88 to 115) should be described separately. Atrial flutter frequently is associated with underlying heart or lung disease.

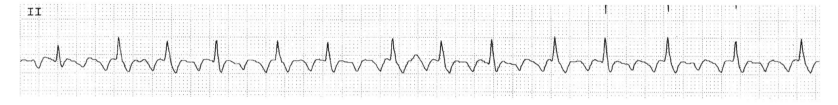

FIGURE 7.6

Premature Atrial Contraction

A premature atrial contraction (PAC) is a premature (too early) ectopic (not from the expected place) beat. A PAC typically throws the rhythm off step, with a slight pause after it. Also, there is a visible P wave right before the PAC. This is called a P′ (P prime) to distinguish it from a normal sinus P wave. PACs can be associated with increased sympathetic activity.

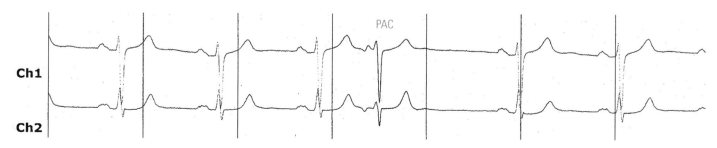

FIGURE 7.7

Sinus Pause

A sinus pause is a period of electrical silence with no activity after a period of sinus rhythm. It is measured in duration from the QRS before the pause to the QRS after the pause, 1.5 seconds in Figure 7.8. Sinus pauses are a sign of underlying disease in the conduction system or a complication of medication such as digitalis, calcium channel blocker, or beta blocker. The most common cause of a sinus pause is a PAC that was nonconducted.

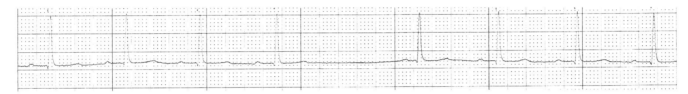

FIGURE 7.8

Atrial Fibrillation

Atrial fibrillation (AF) is an irregularly irregular rhythm. The atrial rhythm may be coarse and visible, or not apparent at all. The ventricular rate is calculated by measuring a 6 second interval, and multiplying the number of QRS complexes by 10. The ventricular rate in Figure 7.9 is 130 bpm. Atrial fibrillation increases in incidence with advancing age. It can be associated with underlying heart diseases such as hypertension, coronary disease, valvular heart disease, and heart failure. It can be associated with acute lung disease such as pulmonary embolism, or chronic lung disease such as COPD. It can be associated with systemic diseases such as hyperthyroidism. It puts the patient at risk for systemic embolism.

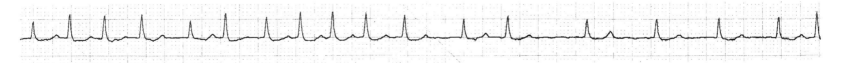

FIGURE 7.9

SAMPLE COMPLETED WORKSHEET

Atrial rate:	Undefined
Ventricular Rate:	40 bpm.
Diagnosis:	Atrial fibrillation

Instructions for Chapter 7 Worksheets

For each arrhythmia, examine the whole strip. Determine an atrial and ventricular rate. In Figure 7.10, the atrial rate in indeterminate. The ventricular rate is irregularly irregular and consistent with atrial fibrillation. The correct way to calculate the heart rate in atrial fibrillation is to count the number of QRS complexes in a random six second sample and then multiply that number by ten to get the ventricular rate in beats per minute (bpm). Figure 7.10 shows 4 QRS complexes in a six-second interval. Four multiplied by ten would yield a ventricular rate of 40 bpm.

Clinical Associations:

Hyperthyroidism, pulmonary embolism, COPD, hypertension, valvular heart disease, CHF

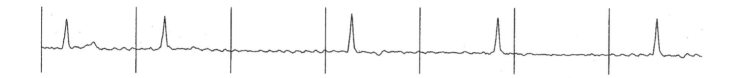

WORKSHEET 7.1

Atrial rate:	
Ventricular Rate:	
Diagnosis:	

Instructions for Chapter 7 Worksheets

For each arrhythmia, examine the whole strip. Determine an atrial and ventricular rate.

Clinical Associations:

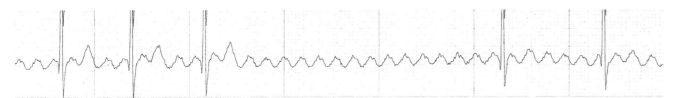

WORKSHEET 7.2

Atrial rate:	
Ventricular Rate:	
Diagnosis:	

Instructions for Chapter 7 Worksheets

For each arrhythmia, examine the whole strip. Determine an atrial and ventricular rate.

Clinical Associations:

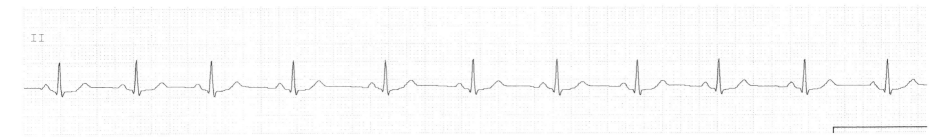

131

WORKSHEET 7.3

Atrial rate:	
Ventricular Rate:	
Diagnosis:	

Instructions for Chapter 7 Worksheets

For each arrhythmia, examine the whole strip. Determine an atrial and ventricular rate.

Clinical Associations:

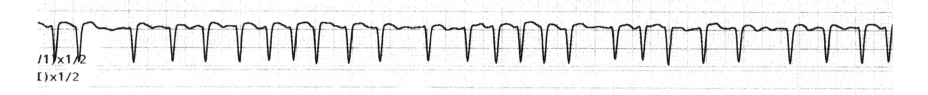

/1)x1/2

[ )x1/2

Ventricular Arrhythmias

Premature Ventricular Contraction

A premature ventricular contraction (PVC) is a single abnormal beat that comes earlier than the expected next beat and is abnormally wide. It originates in the ventricle. The ST segment points away from the QRS in these beats. PVCs occur in normal and abnormal hearts.

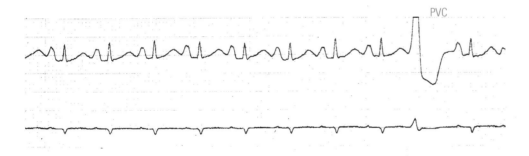

PVC

FIGURE 8.1

Ventricular Bigeminy

PVCs can occur in a pattern that pairs them with a normal beat. **This is called ventricular bigeminy. This can occur in normal and abnormal hearts.**

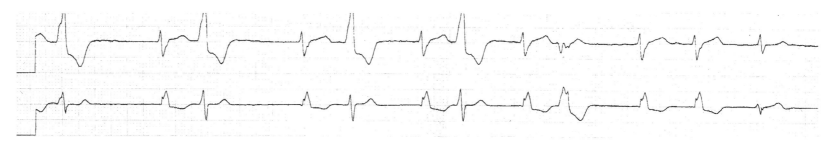

FIGURE 8.2

Ventricular Trigeminy

PVCs can occur in a pattern that pairs them with two normal beats. **This is called ventricular trigeminy, or a trigeminal pattern of PVCs. This can occur in normal and abnormal hearts.**

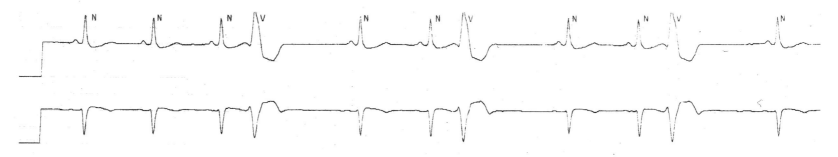

FIGURE 8.3

Paired PVCs

PVCs can occur in pairs, called paired PVCs or coupled PVCs. Paired PVCs have a more unstable rhythm than a single PVC and are more likely to be associated with underlying heart disease than a single PVC. Electrolyte imbalance, particularly hypokalemia, can exacerbate this.

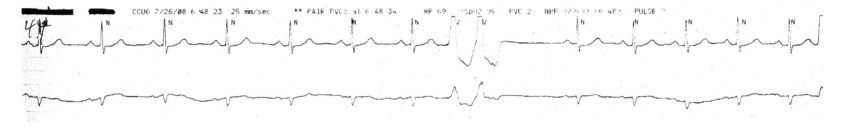

FIGURE 8.4

Ventricular Tachycardia

Ventricular tachycardia (VT) is a regular rhythm originating in the ventricles at a rate of greater than 100 bpm, usually 140 to 260. It has at least three beats. Figure 8.5 demonstrates a self-limited 11-beat episode of VT. VT is usually associated with underlying heart disease, such as coronary disease, cardiomyopathy, hypertension, or congestive heart failure.

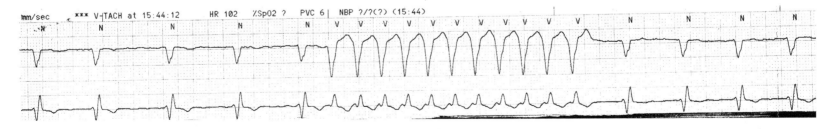

FIGURE 8.5

Ventricular Fibrillation

Ventricular fibrillation (VF) is a fatal arrhythmia that must be rapidly terminated. It is a chaotic electrical discharge that does not effectively depolarize the ventricles and leads to death unless treated effectively and swiftly. It can be seen in acute myocardial ischemia or infarction, congestive heart failure, and cardiomyopathy. Hypokalemia increases the risk of its occurrence.

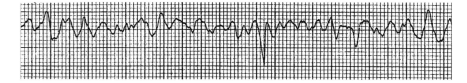

FIGURE 8.6

Artifact

Figure 8.7 demonstrates a rhythm recorded on a two-channel recorder. Both leads are recorded at the exact same time, so any event on the top strip occurs at exactly the same time as an event exactly below it. The rhythm on top appears to be ventricular tachycardia until compared with the bottom strip, which shows sinus rhythm. Manipulation of electrodes can cause this.

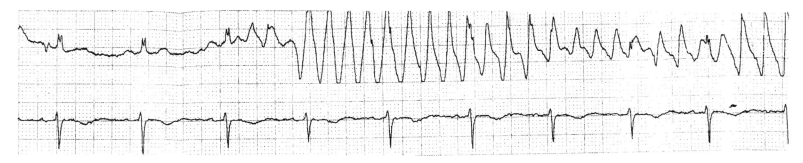

FIGURE 8.7

Torsade de Pointe

Torsade de Pointe (polymophous ventricular tachycardia) is a form of ventricular tachycardia. The diagnostic hallmark of torsade is a change in direction of the complexes. In Figure 8.8, the episode of ventricular tachycardia begins with the first three QRS complexes pointing downward, and the next three pointing upward. This is associated with long QTc interval. Drugs, hypokalemia, and hypocalcemia are common causes.

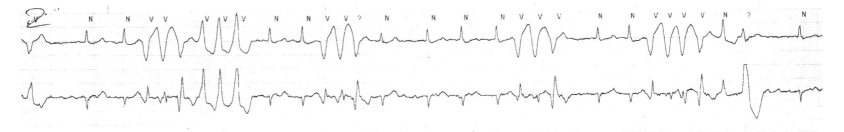

FIGURE 8.8

Idioventricular Rhythm

Idioventricular rhythm is a slow ventricular escape rhythm characterized by wide QRS complexes, typically in a regular slow pattern with no underlying pacing in the ventricles. This is associated with underlying heart disease and can be worsened by beta blockers or calcium channel blockers.

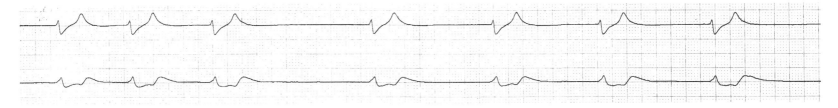

FIGURE 8.9

CHAPTER 8 WORKSHEETS

SAMPLE COMPLETED WORKSHEET

Atrial rate:	Varies
Ventricular Rate:	Ventricular rate: ≥ 100 bpm
Diagnosis:	Paired PVC's, then three beats of Ventricular Tachycardia.

Instructions for Chapter 8 Worksheets

For each arrhythmia, examine the whole strip and determine an atrial and ventricular rate. The P wave samples are not long enough to confirm the underlying rhythm is sinus or to be sure of the underlying atrial rate. The ventricular rate also varies, but is more than 100 beats per minute (bpm). In addition, there is a pair of wide QRS complexes that are premature, making them paired PVCs. This is followed by a sequence of three such beats. This triplet represents ventricular tachycardia, since the QRS complexes are wide and the rate is greater then 100 bpm.

Clinical Associations:

Suspect underlying coronary disease, cardiomyopathy, or CHF. Also consider hypokalemia.

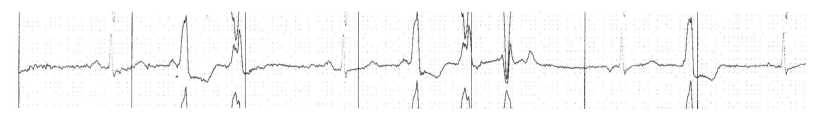

FIGURE 8.10

WORKSHEET 8.1

Atrial rate:	
Ventricular Rate:	
Diagnosis:	

Instructions for Chapter 8 Worksheets

For each arrhythmia, examine the whole strip and determine an atrial and ventricular rate.

Clinical Associations:

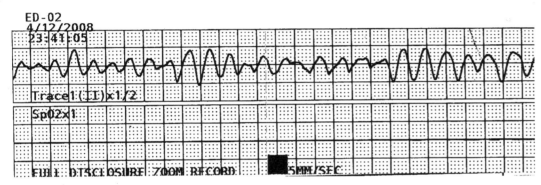

ED-02
4/12/2008
23:41:05

Trace 1 (II) x1/2

SpO2 x1

FULL DISCLOSURE ZOOM RECORD 5MM/SEC

WORKSHEET 8.2

Atrial rate:	
Ventricular Rate:	
Diagnosis:	

Instructions for Chapter 8 Worksheets

For each arrhythmia, examine the whole strip and determine an atrial and ventricular rate.

Clinical Associations:

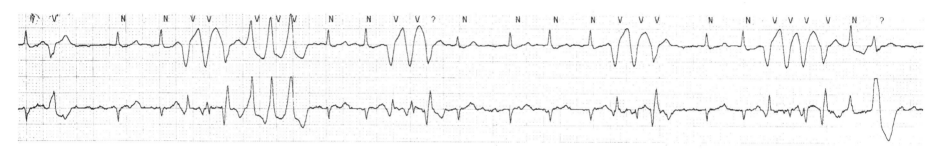

WORKSHEET 8.3

Atrial rate:	
Ventricular Rate:	
Diagnosis:	

Instructions for Chapter 8 Worksheets

For each arrhythmia, examine the whole strip and determine an atrial and ventricular rate.

Clinical Associations:

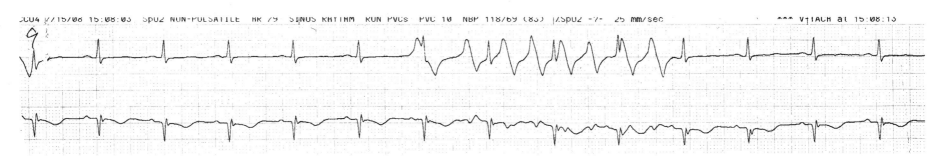

Junctional Rhythm, Heart Block, and Pacemakers

9

Junctional Rhythm

Junctional rhythm is a regular rhythm. A P wave is frequently not seen because the rhythm originates in the AV junctional node. When a P wave is seen, it may precede the QRS, as shown in Figure 9.1 When present, the P wave direction in junctional rhythm is upward. Junctional rhythm may be a manifestation of digitalis toxicity, sick sinus syndrome, and acute inferior wall infarction.

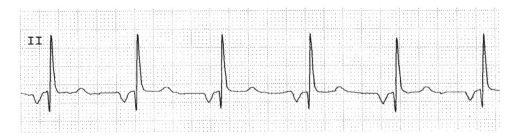

FIGURE 9.1

143

Heart Block

1° AV Block

1° AV block is an abnormally long delay in the transmission of the atrial impulse through the AV node. It causes a prolongation of the PR interval to greater than 0.20 seconds. In Figure 9.2, the PR interval is 0.26 seconds long. Associations include sick sinus syndrome, drugs such as digitalis, calcium channel blockers, and antiarrhythmics.

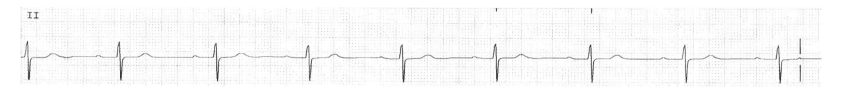

FIGURE 9.2

2° AV Block

2° AV block is a more severe form of conduction abnormality in the AV node. It is characterized by a P wave that "gets lost" in the AV node and never generates a QRS complex on the EKG. There are two types of 2° AV block: Wenckebach (Type I) and Mobitz (Type II). Wenckebach is characterized by an increasing PR interval leading up to a dropped or nonconducted P wave, as shown in Figure 9.3.   Because a grouping of 4 P waves leads to 3 QRS complexes, this is termed 4:3 Wenckebach. Type II (Mobitz) AV block is characterized by sequential P waves (usually more than two) that produce only a single QRS complex.

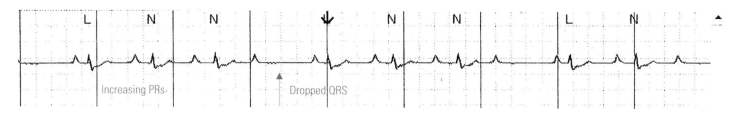

FIGURE 9.3

Premature Atrial Contractions

Pauses are most commonly caused by premature atrial contractions (PACs) that do not conduct down to the ventricle and generate a QRS complex. These are called nonconducted PACs (NCPACs). **Frequently they occur during the T wave, and deform the T wave compared to normal. In Figure 9.4, the premature wave (P′) does not conduct to the ventricles and causes a pause of 2.6 seconds. Nonconducted PACs may be a sign of underlying conduction disease, such as sick sinus syndrome, particularly if they occur late in the cycle and are followed by a long pause.**

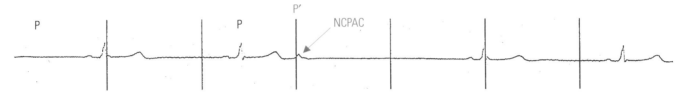

FIGURE 9.4

Sinus Arrest

Asystole is a prolonged period of no electrical activity. In Figure 9.5, for example, a sinus beat is followed by a period of 8 seconds of electrical asystole that continues until the end of the strip. Cessastion of function of the sinus node is called sinus arrest. Normally, when sinus arrest occurs, another pacemaker must take over, such as the junction (usually at an escape rate of 40 to 60 bpm) or the ventricles (usually at an escape rate of 30 bpm). In Figure 9.5, however, there is sinus arrest with no further pacemaker activity anywhere. This leads to asystole, and cardiac arrest.

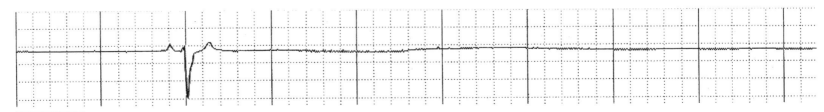

FIGURE 9.5

Complete Heart Block

Complete heart block (CHB), also known as 3° AV block (3° AVB), describes
the presence of atrial activity that does not conduct down to the ventricles
on a continuing basis. Figure 9.6 demonstrates a patient with P waves (P) at a
rate of 83 bpm. The P waves do not generate QRS complexes. A regular ventricular rhythm (V) at a rate of 36 bpm has come in as an escape to provide a
heart beat.

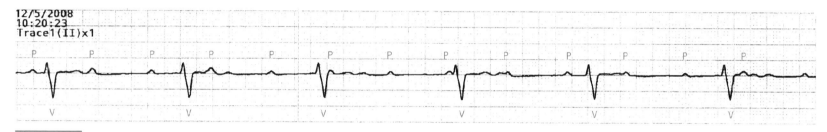

FIGURE 9.6

Ventricular Escape Beats

Ventricular escape beats (VE) are wide QRS complexes that come late and function as a rescue rhythm of last resort for the heart. **They function at a slow rate, usually in the range of 30 to 40 bpm. The ventricular escape mechanism is not as reliable a pacemaker as the sinus node or junction.** It is typically associated with significantly compromised myocardium, as would be seen in cardiac arrest.

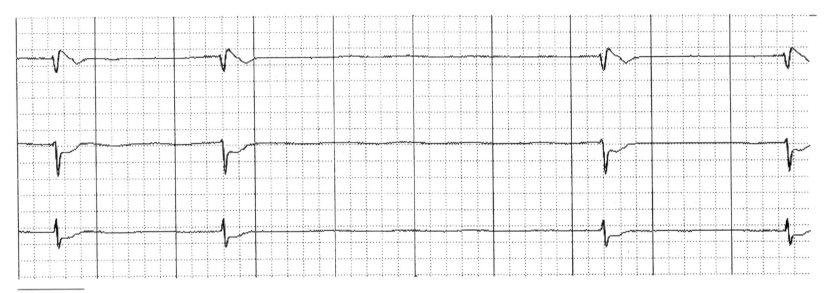

FIGURE 9.7

Asystole

Asystole indicates the total absence of electrical activity. It has the worst prognosis of all cardiac rhythms. In Figure 9.8, the heart is unable to generate even an escape beat from the ventricles to generate a single QRS. The myocardium appears functionally dead.

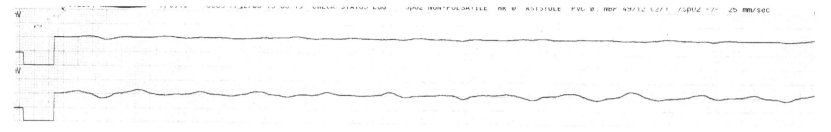

FIGURE 9.8

Pacemakers

Ventricular Pacing

Ventricular pacemaker rhythm demonstrates a vertical electrical artifact (EA) at the beginning of the QRS. Because each QRS in Figure 9.9 begins with a pacing artifact, this is pacemaker rhythm. The presence of the pacing spike (PS) demonstrates pacemaker output. The presence of an ST segment after the QRS proves that the pacemaker captured (depolarized) the ventricles. Ventricular pacemakers are used in the setting of complete heart block or episodes of asytole longer than 3 seconds (off any suspected medications), particularly in the setting of atrial fibrillation.

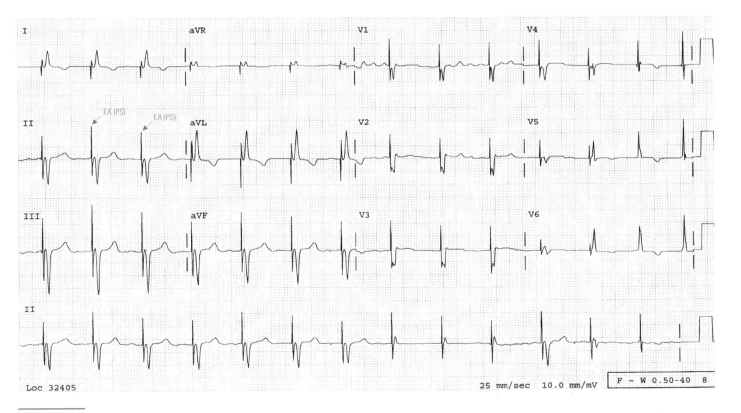

FIGURE 9.9

Ventricular Pacing

Figure 9.10 demonstrates vertical pacing spikes or artifacts before each QRS complex (VPS). In addition, a second pacing spike is present 0.16 seconds before the QRS. This represents an atrial pacing spike (APS). This is called AV sequential pacing. The pacemaker checks that a native beat has not occurred in time. Next it sends a charge into the atrial wall causing atrial depolarization. The pacemaker waits 0.16 seconds acting as an artificial AV node. Finally it sends a second charge into the ventricle depolarizing it. This pacemaker would be used in patients who have heart block or asystole but do not have atrial fibrillation. The use of two-chamber pacing is particularly important in the setting of heart failure.

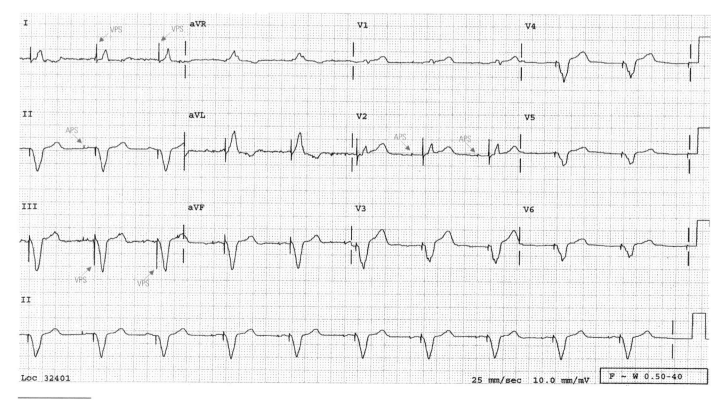

FIGURE 9.10

Atrial Pacing

Figure 9.11 demonstrates atrial pacing alone. The pacemaker waits for the sinus node for a predetermined period of time. After this time passes, the pacemaker sends an electrical charge into the atrium. The rest of conduction is carried out normally through the patient's AV node. Ventricular conduction is through the patient's native conduction system. This system can only be used if the AV node functions normally. It cannot be used in atrial fibrillation.

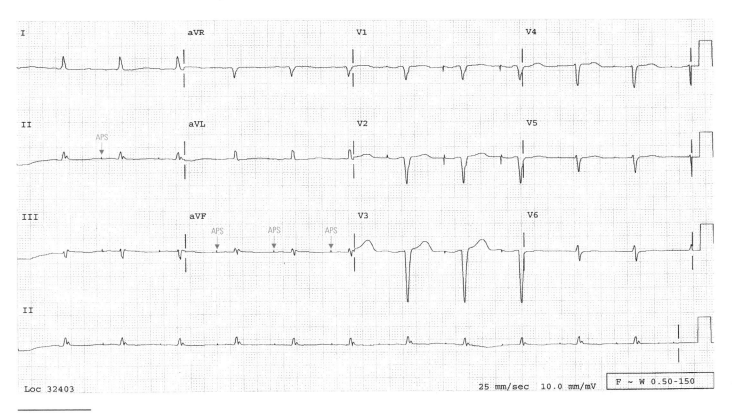

Loc 32403

25 mm/sec   10.0 mm/mV   F ~ W 0.50-150

FIGURE 9.11

WORKSHEET 9.1

Atrial rate:	
Ventricular Rate:	
Diagnosis:	

Instructions for Chapter 9 Worksheets

For each arrhythmia, examine the whole strip and determine an atrial and ventricular rate.

Clinical Associations:

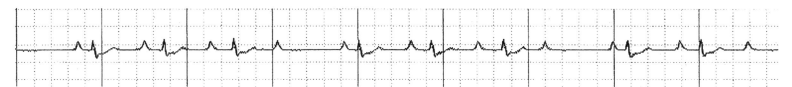

WORKSHEET 9.2

Atrial rate:	
Ventricular Rate:	
Diagnosis:	

Instructions for Chapter 9 Worksheets

For each arrhythmia, examine the whole strip and determine an atrial and ventricular rate.

Clinical Associations:

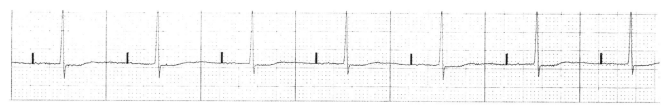

Atrial rate:	
Ventricular Rate:	
Diagnosis:	

Instructions for Chapter 9 Worksheets

For each arrhythmia, examine the whole strip and determine an atrial and ventricular rate.

Clinical Associations:

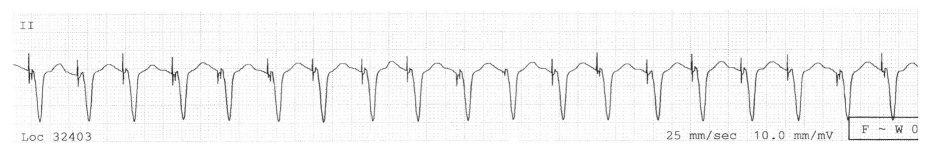

II

Loc 32403   25 mm/sec   10.0 mm/mV   F ~ W 0

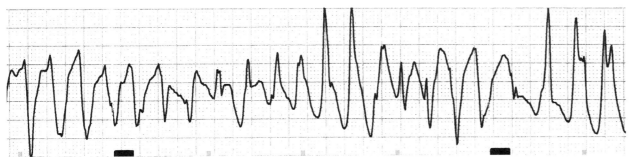

WORKSHEET III.1

Atrial rate:	
Ventricular Rate:	
Diagnosis:	

Instructions for Section III Worksheets

For each arrhythmia, examine the whole strip and determine an atrial and ventricular rate.

Clinical Associations:

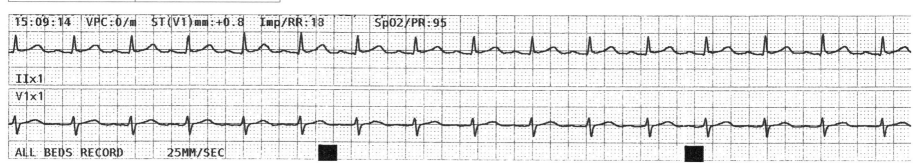

WORKSHEET III.2

Atrial rate:	
Ventricular Rate:	
Diagnosis:	

Instructions for Section III Worksheets

For each arrhythmia, examine the whole strip and determine an atrial and ventricular rate.

Clinical Associations:

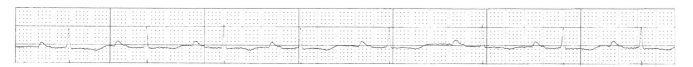

WORKSHEET III.3

Atrial rate:	
Ventricular Rate:	
Diagnosis:	

Instructions for Section III Worksheets

For each arrhythmia, examine the whole strip and determine an atrial and ventricular rate.

Clinical Associations:

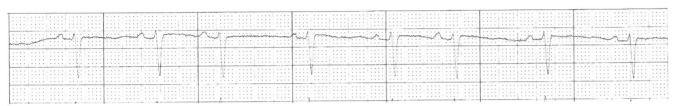

WORKSHEET III.4

Atrial rate:	
Ventricular Rate:	
Diagnosis:	

Instructions for Section III Worksheets

For each arrhythmia, examine the whole strip and determine an atrial and ventricular rate.

Clinical Associations:

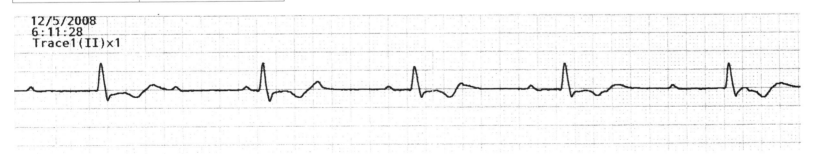

12/5/2008
6:11:28
Trace1(II)x1

WORKSHEET III.5

Atrial rate:	
Ventricular Rate:	
Diagnosis:	

Instructions for Section III Worksheets

For each arrhythmia, examine the whole strip and determine an atrial and ventricular rate.

Clinical Associations:

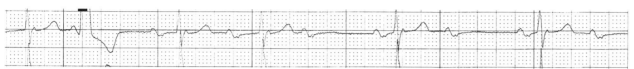

WORKSHEET III.6

Atrial rate:	
Ventricular Rate:	
Diagnosis:	

Instructions for Section III Worksheets

For each arrhythmia, examine the whole strip and determine an atrial and ventricular rate.

Clinical Associations:

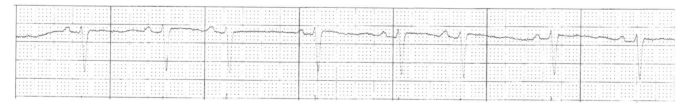

WORKSHEET III.7

Atrial rate:	
Ventricular Rate:	
Diagnosis:	

Instructions for Section III Worksheets

For each arrhythmia, examine the whole strip and determine an atrial and ventricular rate.

Clinical Associations:

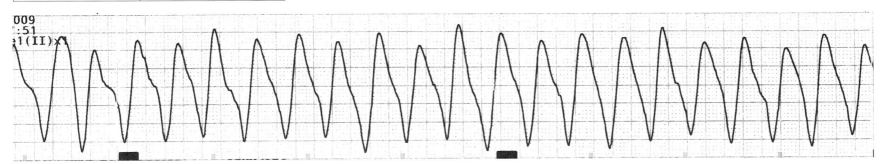

WORKSHEET III.8

Atrial rate:	
Ventricular Rate:	
Diagnosis:	

Instructions for Section III Worksheets

For each arrhythmia, examine the whole strip and determine an atrial and ventricular rate.

Clinical Associations:

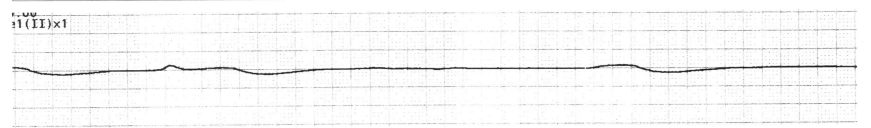

WORKSHEET III.9

Atrial rate:	
Ventricular Rate:	
Diagnosis:	

Instructions for Section III Worksheets

For each arrhythmia, examine the whole strip and determine an atrial and ventricular rate.

Clinical Associations:

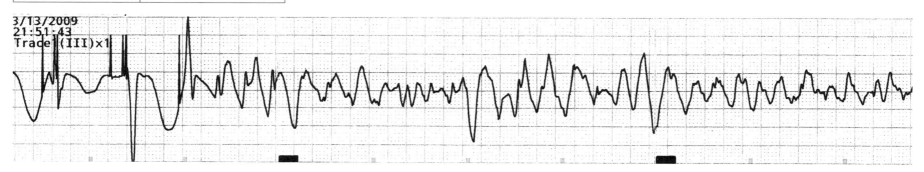

3/13/2009
21:51:43
Trace (III)×1

WORKSHEET III.10

Atrial rate:	
Ventricular Rate:	
Diagnosis:	

Instructions for Section III Worksheets

For each arrhythmia, examine the whole strip and determine an atrial and ventricular rate.

Clinical Associations:

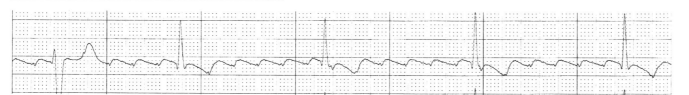

WORKSHEET III.11

Atrial rate:	
Ventricular Rate:	
Diagnosis:	

Instructions for Section III Worksheets

For each arrhythmia, examine the whole strip and determine an atrial and ventricular rate.

Clinical Associations:

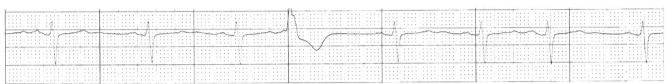

WORKSHEET III.12

Atrial rate:	
Ventricular Rate:	
Diagnosis:	

Instructions for Section III Worksheets

For each arrhythmia, examine the whole strip and determine an atrial and ventricular rate.

Clinical Associations:

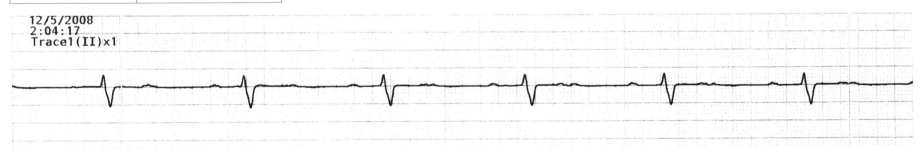

12/5/2008
2:04:17
Trace1(II)x1

WORKSHEET III.13

Atrial rate:	
Ventricular Rate:	
Diagnosis:	

Instructions for Section III Worksheets

For each arrhythmia, examine the whole strip and determine an atrial and ventricular rate.

Clinical Associations:

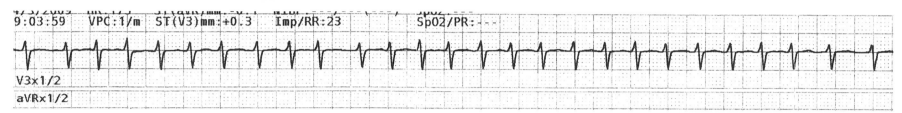

WORKSHEET III.14

Atrial rate:	
Ventricular Rate:	
Diagnosis:	

Instructions for Section III Worksheets

For each arrhythmia, examine the whole strip and determine an atrial and ventricular rate.

Clinical Associations:

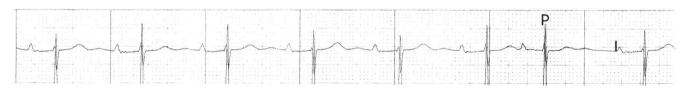

Atrial rate:	
Ventricular Rate:	
Diagnosis:	

Instructions for Section III Worksheets

For each arrhythmia, examine the whole strip and determine an atrial and ventricular rate.

Clinical Associations:

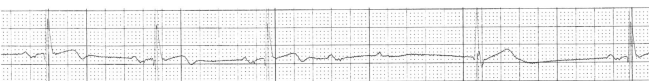

EKG Changes
Related to Conduction
Abnormalities

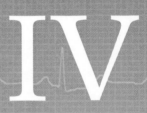

IV

Hemiblock

Self-Study Objectives

- ▦ Identify the components of the conduction system
- ▦ Identify the two parts of the left bundle
- ▦ Describe the criteria for left anterior hemiblock
- ▦ Describe the criteria for left posterior hemiblock
- ▦ Identify left anterior hemiblock on the EKG
- ▦ Identify left posterior hemiblock on the EKG

Overview

The heart has specialized cells that enable the five critical electrical and mechanical functions. The sinus node established the first of the five critical functions—the ability to create an automatic and regular heart rhythm. The second critical function allows for communication between billions of cells in less than one or two tenths of a second. This conduction system is an exquisitely capable communication system. It carefully navigates the impulse from the atria through the normal AV node and the bundle of His, then through the right and left bundles and the Purkinje fibers, before finally depolarizing every single one of the billions of ventricular cells. The right and left bundles are directly responsible for conducting, or communicating, the electrical signal to all cells in both ventricles (Figure 10.1).

The Left Bundle Branch

The left bundle has two parts (sometimes called fascicles) that help it communicate with the far greater number of cells in the left ventricle. The parts are called the anterior and posterior divisions, which are responsible for depolarization of the left ventricle, including the septum. Hemiblock is the loss of function in one of the two parts of the left bundle (Figure 10.2).

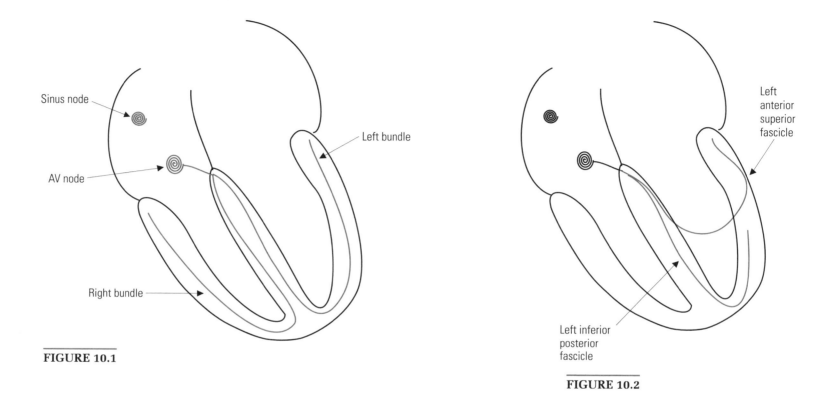

FIGURE 10.1

FIGURE 10.2

Left Anterior Hemiblock: Pathophysiology

Left anterior hemiblock (LAHB) occurs when there is a loss of function in the anterior branch or fascicle of the left bundle branch (Figure 10.3). It is diagnosed by evaluating the mean QRS axis, or direction, in the frontal plane. The normal QRS direction is from the AV node toward the apex of the heart, that is inferiorly and to the patient's left side. Left anterior hemiblock shifts the mean QRS axis upward and leftward (Figure 10.4). This occurs because the electrical impulse from the left inferior fascicle spreads superiorly and to the left to depolarize the entire left ventricle since the left anterior branch is unable to do so. Left anterior hemiblock is sometimes called left anterior superior hemiblock (LASH), which calls attention to the diagnostic trademark of LAHB, namely a superior QRS direction in the frontal plane. The two terms are synonymous. Of note, hemiblock does not significantly increase the duration of the QRS interval because each side of the heart has one functioning fascicle.

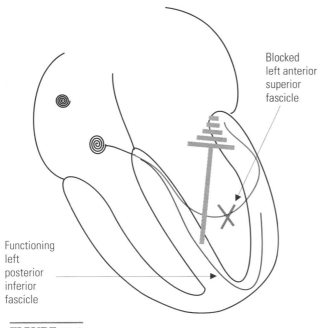

Blocked
left anterior
superior
fascicle

Functioning
left
posterior
inferior
fascicle

FIGURE 10.3

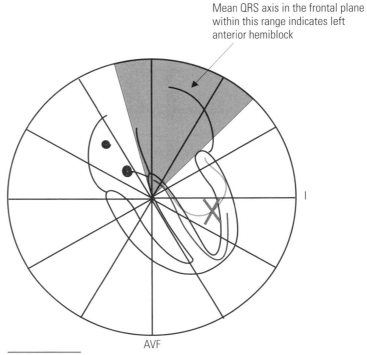

Mean QRS axis in the frontal plane
within this range indicates left
anterior hemiblock

I

AVF

FIGURE 10.4

Left Anterior Hemiblock: Criteria

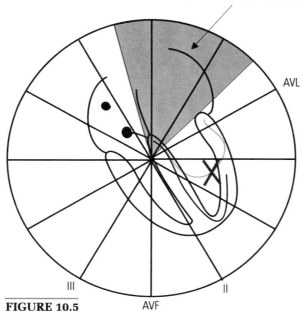

Mean QRS direction in the frontal plane within this range indicates left anterior hemiblock

AVL

I

III

II

AVF

FIGURE 10.5

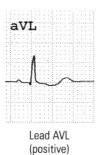

Lead AVL
(positive)

FIGURE 10.6a

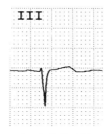

Leads II, III, AFV
(negative)

FIGURE 10.6b

Left Anterior Hemiblock: Step-by-Step Example

a) Lead I is positive, so the QRS direction is to the patient's left side (somewhere between −90 and +90).

b) Lead AVF is negative, so the QRS direction is upward (this narrows it down to between 0 and −90).

c) Lead II is negative, so the QRS direction is more negative than −30 (this narrows it down to between −30 and −90).

d) Lead AVR is negative, so the QRS direction is more positive than −60. Thus the QRS is between −30 and −60, or −45!

e) We visualize the QRS direction in the frontal plane as pointing towards the patient's left shoulder. This is the diagnostic characteristic of LAHB.

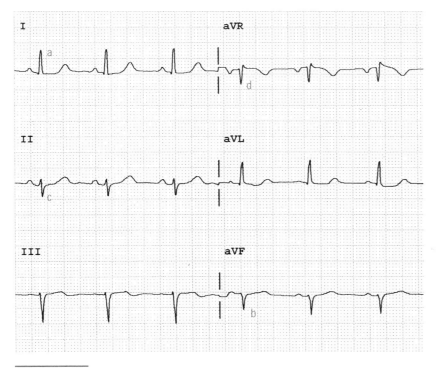

FIGURE 10.7

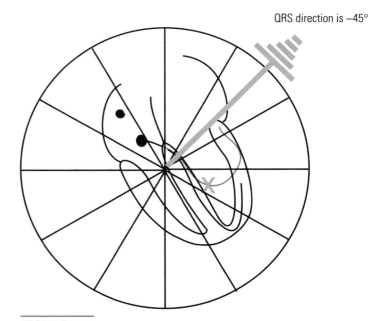

QRS direction is −45°

FIGURE 10.8

Left Posterior Hemiblock: Pathophysiology

The second type of hemiblock is called left posterior hemiblock (LPHB). It occurs when there is a loss of function in the posterior part or fascicle of the left bundle branch. Like LAHB, it is diagnosed by evaluating the mean QRS axis or direction in the frontal plane. The normal QRS direction is from the AV node toward the apex of the heart, that is inferiorly and to the patient's left side. Left posterior hemiblock shifts the mean QSR axis to the patient's right side. This occurs because the electrical impulse from the left anterior fascicle spreads inferiorly and to the right to depolarize the entire left ventricle since

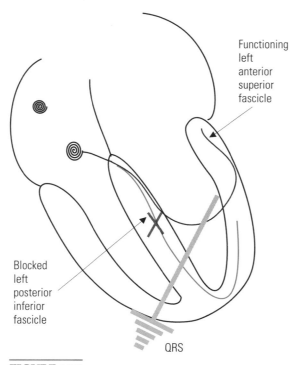

Functioning left anterior superior fascicle

Blocked left posterior inferior fascicle

QRS

FIGURE 10.9

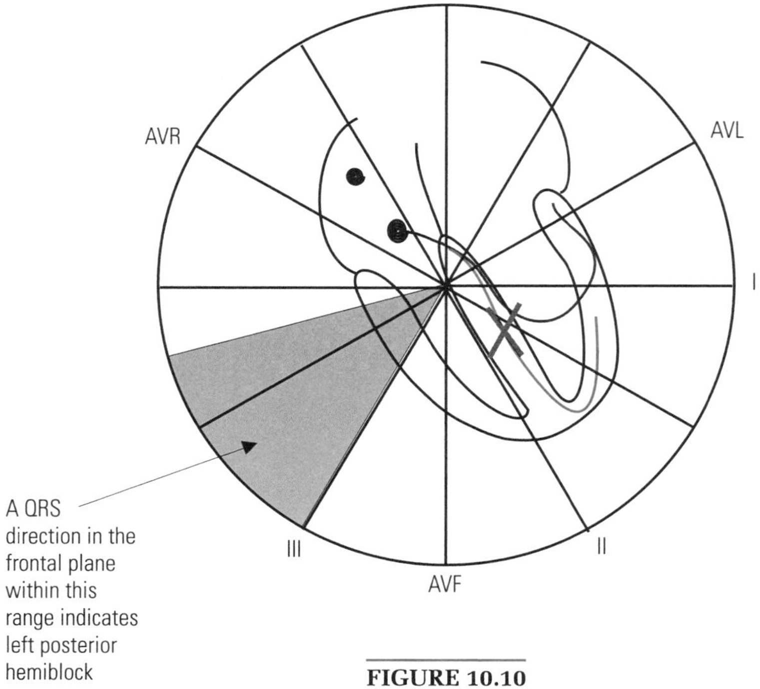

AVR

AVL

I

III

II

AVF

A QRS direction in the frontal plane within this range indicates left posterior hemiblock

FIGURE 10.10

the left posterior branch is unable to do so. Left posterior hemiblock is sometimes called left inferior posterior hemiblock (LIPH), which calls attention to the diagnostic trademark of LIPH, namely an inferior and rightward QRS direction in the frontal plane. The two terms are synonymous. Again, hemiblock does not significantly increase the duration of the QRS interval since each side of the heart has one functioning fascicle.

Left Posterior Hemiblock: Criteria

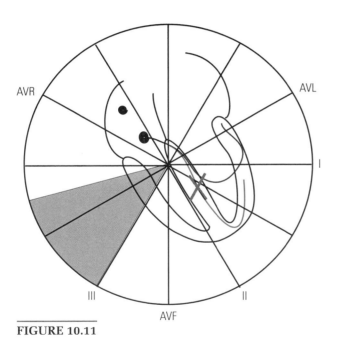

FIGURE 10.11

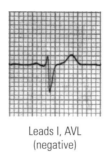

Leads I, AVL
(negative)

FIGURE 10.12a

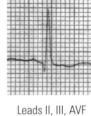

Leads II, III, AVF
(positive)

FIGURE 10.12b

Left Posterior Hemiblock: Step-by-Step Example (Figure 10.13)

a) Lead I is negative, so the QRS direction is to the patient's right side (somewhere more negative than −90, or more positive than +90).
b) Lead AVF is positive, so the QRS direction is downward (this narrows it down to between +90 and +180).
c) Lead II is positive, so the QRS direction is less than +150 (this narrows it down to between +90 and +150).
d) Lead AVR is close to isoelectric, so the QRS direction is perpendicular to it. Thus the QRS is either −60 or +120!
e) We visualize the QRS direction in the frontal plane as pointing towards the patient's right foot. This is the diagnostic characteristic of LPHB.

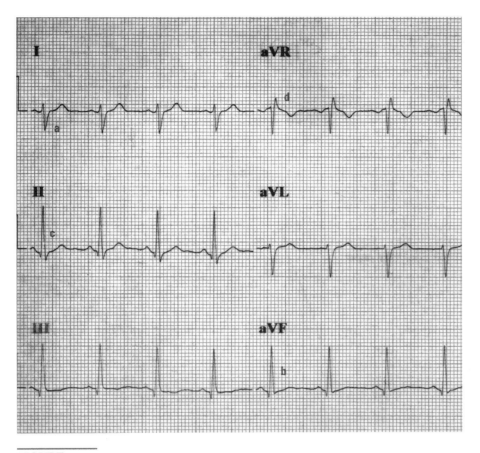

FIGURE 10.13

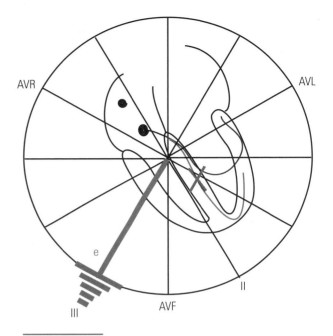

FIGURE 10.14

SAMPLE COMPLETED WORKSHEET

BASIC MEASUREMENTS

Parameter	Measurement	Interpretation
HR	120	Abnormal
Rhythm	Sinus Tach	Abnormal
PR	0.12	Normal
QRS	0.08	Normal
QT	0.30	
QTc	0.44	Long
P direction	Inferior and leftward	Normal
QRS direction	Superior, -45^0	LAHB

Instructions for Chapter 10 Worksheets

A) Complete basic measurements
B) Describe (or caluculate!) the QRS direction in the frontal plane as inferior and left, superior, or rightward.
C) Clinically Diagnose LAHB if the QRS direction is superior. Diagnose LPHB if the QRS direction is inferior and rightward.

Clinically Based Critical Interpretation

Left anterior Hemiblock is present based on the QRS direction pointing superiorly. By itself, LAHB does not have any specific clinical associations other than the presence of conduction disease. Sinus tachycardia is present and should be explained.

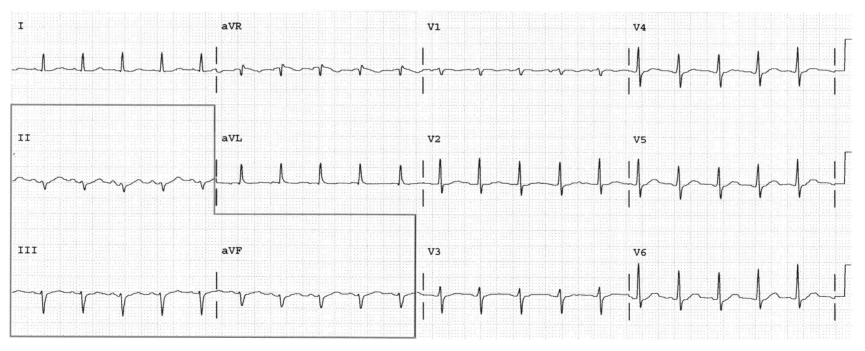

BASIC MEASUREMENTS

Parameter	Measurement	Interpretation
HR		
Rhythm		
PR		
QRS		
QT		
QTc		
P direction		
QRS direction		

Instructions for Chapter 10 Worksheets

A) Complete basic measurements
B) Describe (or caluculate!) the QRS direction in the frontal plane as inferior and left, superior, or rightward.
C) Clinically Diagnose LAHB if the QRS direction is superior. Diagnose LPHB if the QRS direction is inferior and rightward.

Clinically Based Critical Thinking: Interpretation

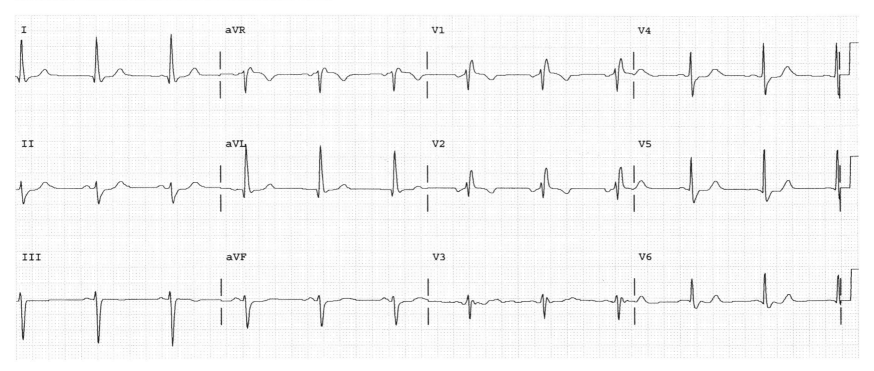

BASIC MEASUREMENTS		
Parameter	**Measurement**	**Interpretation**
HR		
Rhythm		
PR		
QRS		
QT		
QTc		
P direction		
QRS direction		

Instructions for Chapter 10 Worksheets

A) Complete basic measurements
B) Describe (or caluculate!) the QRS direction in the frontal plane as inferior and left, superior, or rightward.
C) Clinically Diagnose LAHB if the QRS direction is superior. Diagnose LPHB if the QRS direction is inferior and rightward.

Clinically Based Critical Thinking: Interpretation

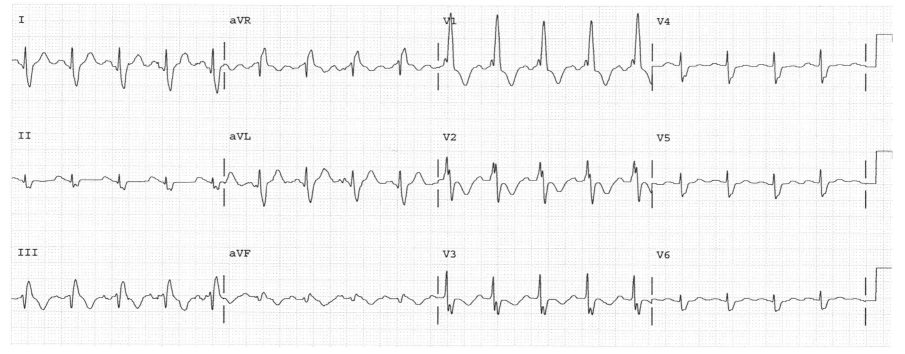

BASIC MEASUREMENTS		
Parameter	Measurement	Interpretation
HR		
Rhythm		
PR		
QRS		
QT		
QTc		
P direction		
QRS direction		

Instructions for Chapter 10 Worksheets

A) Complete basic measurements
B) Describe (or caluculate!) the QRS direction in the frontal plane as inferior and left, superior, or rightward.
C) Clinically Diagnose LAHB if the QRS direction is superior. Diagnose LPHB if the QRS direction is inferior and rightward.

Clinically Based Critical Thinking: Interpretation

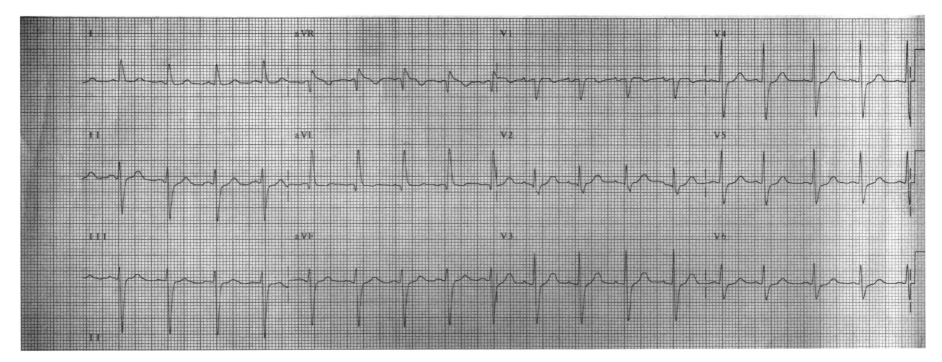

Right Bundle Branch Block

Normal Physiology of QRS Formation

The heart has specialized cells that enable the five critical electrical and mechanical functions. The sinus node established the first of the five critical functions—the ability to create an automatic and regular heart rhythm. The AV node established the second critical function—the ability to delay and then conduct the electrical impulse between the atrium and the ventricle. The right and left bundles provide the third function—communication of the impulse to billions of cells in the right and left ventricles to provide for nearly simultaneous activation of both ventricles. The right and left bundles form an exquisitely capable communication system. They carefully navigate the impulse and depolarize every single one of the billions of ventricular cells. This depolarization of the right and left ventricles forms the normal QRS with a normal interval of 0.08 (Figure 11.1).

Self-Study Objectives: Electrocardiograms

- Define and identify the following:
  Normal QRS interval
  Normal QRS direction
- Define the two EKG criteria for RBBB
- Recognize RBBB in the presence of
  No other disease
  Hemiblock
  Myocardial infarction
- Describe the expected ST changes in RBBB

Learning Objectives: Clinically Based Critical Interpretation

- Define the pathophysiology of
  Right bundle branch block
- Describe the prognosis of right bundle branch block

179

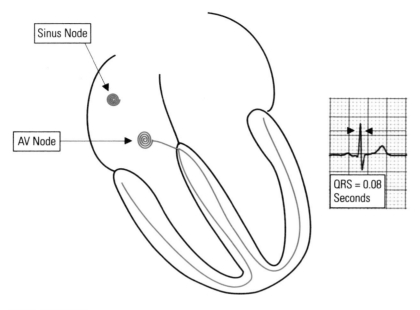

FIGURE 11.1

Normal QRS Physiology Visualized

The normal QRS complex **represents combined depolarization of all the right and left ventricular cells. This normally happens, from first cell to last, in 0.08 seconds. The message to depolarize is conducted to both the right ventricle and left ventricle.** The normal direction of the QRS, as was discussed in Chapters 6 and 11, is toward the left ventricle apex, inferiorly and to the left. This is because the left ventricle has more mass than the right ventricle. This bigger mass creates a bigger electrical force on the EKG than the smaller right ventricle. **Both ventricles normally depolarize at the same time, and so the left ventricular component of the total electrical force overshadows the much smaller right ventricular force. In the frontal view, the QRS points to the patient's left side, which is upward in lead I. In the horizontal view (from above), the direction of the QRS points posteriorly, which is negative in lead V2. (Review Figure 6.63)**

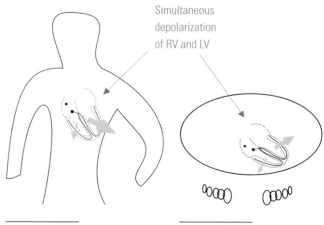

FIGURE 11.2　　**FIGURE 11.3**

Right Bundle Branch Block: Pathophysiology

In right bundle branch block, this all changes. The ventricles are not depolarized at the same time, but in sequence—first the left ventricle, then the right ventricle. The sequence begins with the left bundle, since it is functioning normally. It depolarizes the whole left ventricle in the normal amount of time, which is less than 0.10 seconds. The rest of the QRS after that first 0.08 seconds represents only right ventricular activation. (The whole left ventricle was finished depolarizing in the first 0.08 seconds.) This is the second part of the sequence, depolarization of the right ventricle from the efforts of the left bundle. Since the depolarization of both ventricles is not simultaneous but sequential, it takes longer to finish, 50% longer to finish compared with the normal QRS of 0.08 seconds. Prolongation of the QRS interval to 0.12 seconds or more is the diagnostic signature of bundle branch block. This sequential depolarization allows for the second hallmark of RBBB, namely, that the last part of the depolarization sequence (the QRS) must be right ventricular in direction. In RBBB, the left bundle finishes off ventricular activation on the right side, so the QRS ends in the right ventricle, a direction that is rightward and anterior.

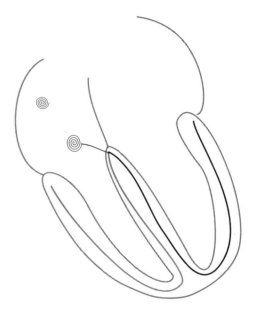

FIGURE 11.4

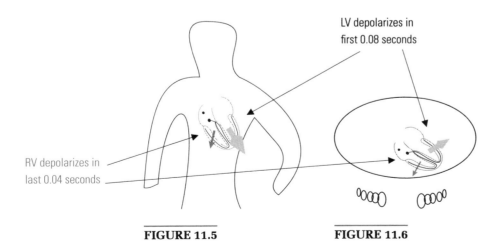

LV depolarizes in first 0.08 seconds

RV depolarizes in last 0.04 seconds

FIGURE 11.5   **FIGURE 11.6**

Right Bundle Branch Block: EKG in the Frontal Plane

Prolongation of the QRS interval to 0.12 seconds or more is the diagnostic signature of bundle branch block. This sequential depolarization allows for the second hallmark of RBBB, namely, that the last part of the depolarization sequence (the QRS) must be right ventricular in direction. In RBBB, ventricular activation finishes on the right side, so the QRS ends in the right ventricle, a direction that is toward the patient's right side and anterior. When the QRS interval is 0.12 seconds or more, bundle branch block is present. Visualize the direction of the end of the QRS in lead I. Since it is negative, it points to the right ventricle and RBBB is present.

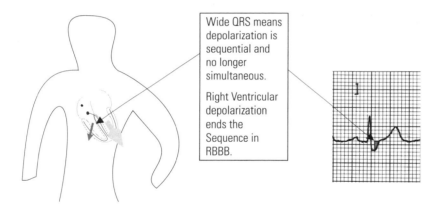

Wide QRS means depolarization is sequential and no longer simultaneous.

Right Ventricular depolarization ends the Sequence in RBBB.

FIGURE 11.7

Right Bundle Branch Block: EKG in the Horizontal Plane

Prolongation of the QRS interval to 0.12 seconds or more is the diagnostic signature of bundle branch block. **This sequential depolarization allows for the second hallmark of RBBB, namely, that** the last part of the depolarization sequence (the QRS) must be right ventricular in direction. **In RBBB, ventricular activation finishes on the right side, so the QRS ends in the right ventricle, a direction that is toward the patient's right side and anterior. When the QRS interval is 0.12 seconds or more, bundle branch block is present.** Visualize the direction of the end of the QRS in lead V1. Since it is positive, it points to the right ventricle, and RBBB is present.

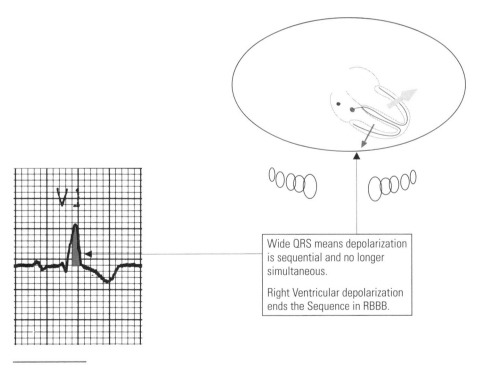

Wide QRS means depolarization is sequential and no longer simultaneous.

Right Ventricular depolarization ends the Sequence in RBBB.

FIGURE 11.8

Right Bundle Branch Block: Summary of Criteria

Criteria 1: The QRS interval is 0.12 seconds or longer
Criteria 2: The last part of the QRS is moving toward the right ventricle, which is right and anterior.
  A) Limb Leads: The QRS ends in an S wave in Lead I, and in V6. This is a rightward direction (Figure 11.9)
  B) Horizontal Leads: The QRS ends in an R or R′ wave in Lead V1. This is an anterior and rightward direction (Figure 11.10)
Critical Point: The first half of the QRS is irrelevant in making the diagnosis of RBBB!

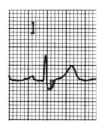
FIGURE 11.9

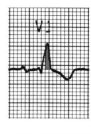
FIGURE 11.10

Right Bundle Branch Block: Abnormal ST Segments

In RBBB the ST segment is predictably abnormal and points away from the right ventricle. In Figure 11.11, the last part of the QRS is negative in lead I, so the ST segment should point away from this, or manifest ST segment elevation in that lead. In lead V1 (Figure 11.12), the last part of the QRS is positive, so the ST segment should point away from that, or manifest ST segment depression. In RBBB, the formation of the QRS is sequential. Because of this, do not diagnose right ventricular hypertrophy in the setting of RBBB. All other parts of the EKG, particularly hemiblock, ischemia, and infarction, can be diagnosed and should be evaluated.

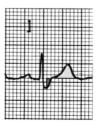

In Right Bundle Branch Block, expect the ST segment to point in the opposite direction from the last part of the QRS.

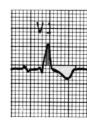

FIGURE 11.11

FIGURE 11.12

Right Bundle Branch Block: Example 1

This is an example of the simple case of RBBB. It meets the two criteria for diagnosis. First, the QRS interval is 0.12 seconds or more. This means the ventricles were not depolarized simultaneously, but in sequence. Since the ventricles are out of sequence, inspection of the last half of the QRS identifies the late or delayed ventricle. In Figure 11.13, the end of the QRS in lead I is an S wave, and so points rightward. The end of the QRS in lead V1 is positive, and so points anteriorly and rightward. In both leads I and V1, the delayed part of the QRS points to the right ventricle. Since the right ventricle is delayed, it must be the right bundle that is blocked.

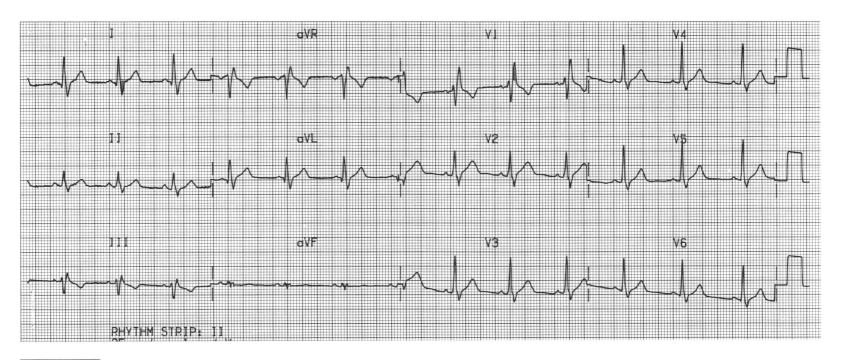

FIGURE 11.13

Right Bundle Branch Block with Hemiblock: Example 2

This is an example of RBBB with associated hemiblock. First, the QRS interval is 0.12 seconds or more. This is the diagnostic hallmark of bundle branch block. This means the ventricles were not depolarized simultaneously, but sequentially. Since the ventricles are out of sequence, inspection of the last half of the QRS again identifies the late or delayed ventricle. In Figure 11.14, the end of the QRS in lead I is an S wave, and so points rightward. The end of the QRS in lead V1 is positive, and so points anteriorly and rightward. In both leads I and V1, the delayed part of the QRS points to the right ventricle. Since the right ventricle is delayed, it must be the right bundle that is blocked.

Remember, only the END of the QRS is used to diagnose bundle branch block. To determine if hemiblock is also present, the ENTIRE QRS is evaluated and visualized to determine its direction. Right bundle branch block does not alter the overall direction of the QRS, which should still be pointing inferiorly and to the patient's left side. In this example the whole QRS points upward (since it is negative in leads II, III and AVF—mathematically it is –75 degrees). Therefore, the EKG in Figure 11.14 has LAHB as well. The same criteria apply for diagnosing hemiblock whether or not RBBB is present. Always check for the presence of hemiblock when RBBB is detected.

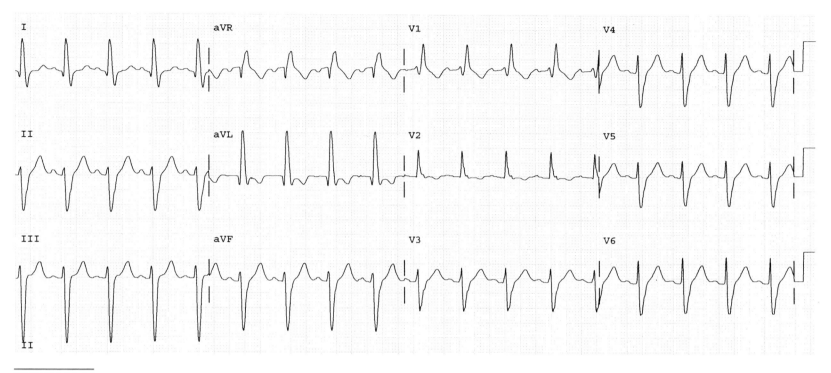

FIGURE 11.14

Right Bundle Branch Block with Anterior Infarction: Example 3

RBBB can be associated with infarction of the anterior wall (see Chapter 15). The criteria for RBBB remain unaffected by the presence of infarction or hemiblock. First, the QRS interval in Figure 11.15 is 0.12 seconds or more. This is the diagnostic hallmark of bundle branch block. Again, this means the ventricles were not depolarized simultaneously, but sequentially. Since the ventricles are out of sequence, inspection of the last half of the QRS again identifies the late or delayed ventricle. In Figure 11.15, the end of the QRS in lead I is an S wave, and so points rightward. The end of the QRS in lead V1 is positive, and so points anteriorly and rightward. In both leads I and V1 the delayed part of the QRS points to the right ventricle. Since the right ventricle is delayed, it must be the right bundle that is blocked. Using a step-by-step approach, the diagnosis of RBBB in the presence of infarction or hemiblock is straightforward.

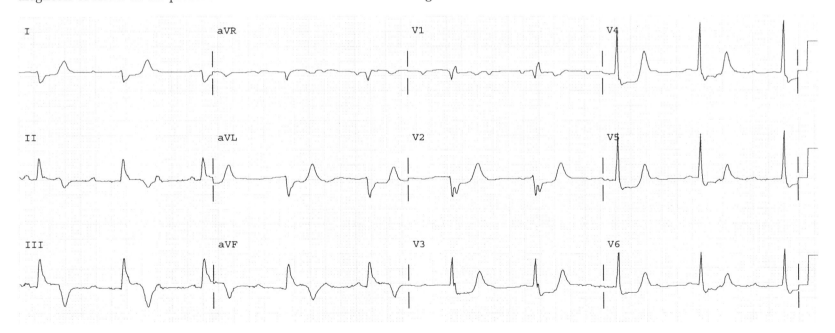

FIGURE 11.15

Incomplete Right Bundle Branch Block: Pathophysiology

Less than total loss of function in either the right or left bundle is called intraventricular conduction delay (IVCD) or incomplete RBBB. The primary diagnostic EKG abnormality in IVCD is prolongation of the QRS interval to 0.10 or 0.11 seconds. As in bundle branch block, IVCD may be left, right, or indeterminate. Once the QRS interval is measured at 0.10 or 0.11 seconds, it is the end of the QRS that is the key to diagnosis. If the end of the QRS is rightward (negative in lead I) and toward the right ventricle (positive in lead V1), then RIVCD is present.

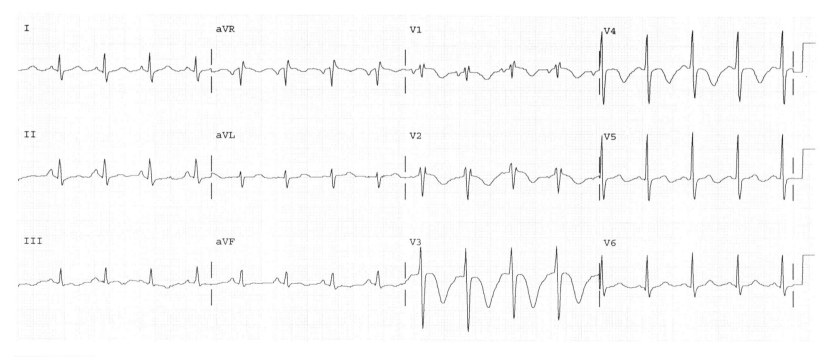

FIGURE 11.16

SAMPLE COMPLETED WORKSHEET

BASIC MEASUREMENTS

Parameter	Measurement	Interpretation
HR	79	Normal
Rhythm	Sinus	Normal
PR	0.12	Normal
QRS	0.13	RBBB
QT	0.36	
QTc	0.40	Normal
P direction	Inferior and leftward	Normal
QRS direction	Superior	LAHB

Instructions for Chapter 11 Worksheets

A) Complete basic measurements.
B) If the QRS is ≥ 0.12 sec, diagnose BBB. Then visualize the extra piece at the end of the QRS in the frontal plane as right or left, and in the horizontal plane as anterior or posterior. Diagnose BBB further as RBBB if the end of the QRS points to the right ventricle (rightward and anteriorly). Always look for hemiblock, which may be present as well. The criteria for the diagnosis of hemiblock do not change when RBBB is present.
C) Provide an interpretation.

Clinically Based Critical Thinking: Interpretation

RBBB are LAHB are both diseases of the conduction system. The combination does not have a significant clinical correlation. The added presence of either 1°AV Block (which is not present on this EKG), or symptoms of syncope would suggest the presence of further conduction disease.

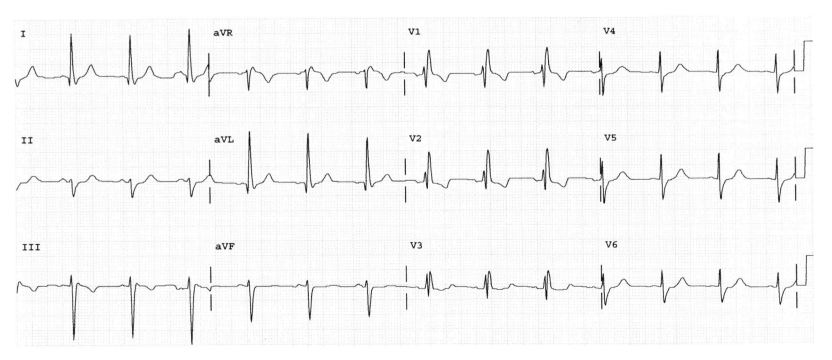

BASIC MEASUREMENTS		
Parameter	Measurement	Interpretation
HR		
Rhythm		
PR		
QRS		
QT		
QTc		
P direction		
QRS direction		

Instructions for Chapter 11 Worksheets

A) Complete basic measurements.

B) If the QRS is ≥ 0.12 sec, diagnose BBB. Then visualize the extra piece at the end of the QRS in the frontal plane as right or left, and in the horizontal plane as anterior or posterior. Diagnose BBB further as RBBB if the end of the QRS points to the right ventricle (rightward and anteriorly). Always look for hemiblock, which may be present as well. The criteria for the diagnosis of hemiblock do not change when RBBB is present.

C) Provide an interpretation.

Clinically Based Critical Thinking: Interpretation

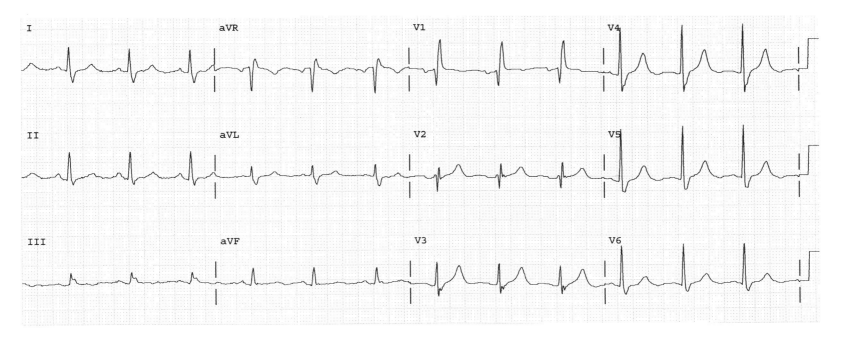

BASIC MEASUREMENTS		
Parameter	**Measurement**	**Interpretation**
HR		
Rhythm		
PR		
QRS		
QT		
QTc		
P direction		
QRS direction		

Instructions for Chapter 11 Worksheets

A) Complete basic measurements.
B) If the QRS is ≥ 0.12 sec, diagnose BBB. Then visualize the extra piece at the end of the QRS in the frontal plane as right or left, and in the horizontal plane as anterior or posterior. Diagnose BBB further as RBBB if the end of the QRS points to the right ventricle (rightward and anteriorly). Always look for hemiblock, which may be present as well. The criteria for the diagnosis of hemiblock do not change when RBBB is present.
C) Provide an interpretation.

Clinically Based Critical Thinking: Interpretation

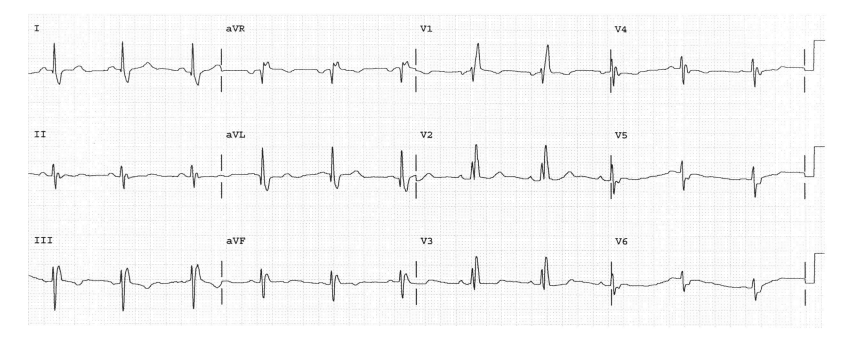

WORKSHEET 11.3

BASIC MEASUREMENTS		
Parameter	Measurement	Interpretation
HR		
Rhythm		
PR		
QRS		
QT		
QTc		
P direction		
QRS direction		

Instructions for Chapter 11 Worksheets

A) Complete basic measurements.
B) If the QRS is ≥ 0.12 sec, diagnose BBB. Then visualize the extra piece at the end of the QRS in the frontal plane as right or left, and in the horizontal plane as anterior or posterior. Diagnose BBB further as RBBB if the end of the QRS points to the right ventricle (rightward and anteriorly). Always look for hemiblock, which may be present as well. The criteria for the diagnosis of hemiblock do not change when RBBB is present.
C) Provide an interpretation.

Clinically Based Critical Thinking: Interpretation

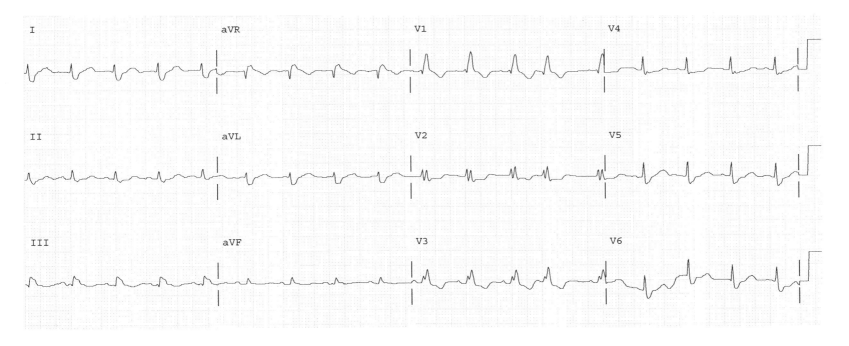

Left Bundle Branch Block

Normal Physiology of QRS Formation

The heart has specialized cells that enable the five critical electrical and mechanical functions. The sinus node established the first of the five critical functions—the ability to create an automatic and regular heart rhythm. The AV node established the second critical function—the ability to delay and then conduct the electrical impulse between the atrium and the ventricle. The right and left bundles provide the third function—communication of the impulse to billions of cells in the right and left ventricles to provide for nearly simultaneous activation of both ventricles. The right and left bundles (Figure 12.1) form an exquisitely capable communication system. They carefully navigate the impulse and depolarize every single one of the billions of ventricular cells. This depolarization of the right and left ventricles forms the normal QRS with a normal interval of 0.08 (Figure 12.2).

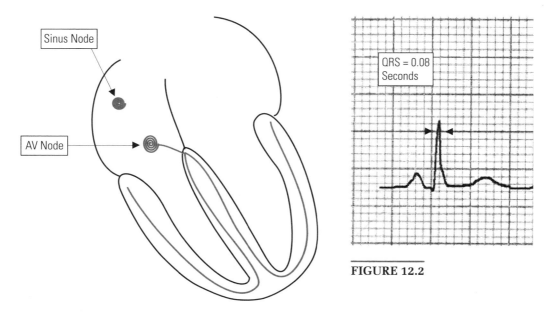

Sinus Node

AV Node

QRS = 0.08 Seconds

FIGURE 12.2

FIGURE 12.1

Normal QRS Physiology Visualized: Frontal Plane

The normal QRS complex represents combined depolarization of all the right and left ventricular cells (Figure 12.2). This normally happens, from first cell to last, in 0.08 seconds. The message to depolarize is conducted to both the right ventricle and left ventricle. The normal direction of the QRS (as was discussed in Chapters 6 and 11) is toward the left ventricle apex, inferiorly and to the left. This is because the left ventricle has more mass than the right ventricle. This bigger mass creates a bigger electrical force on the EKG than the smaller right ventricle. Both ventricles normally depolarize at the same time, and so the left ventricular component of the total electrical force overshadows the much smaller right ventricular force. In the frontal view, the QRS points to the patient's left side, which is upward in lead I. In the horizontal view (from above), the direction of the QRS points posteriorly, which is negative in lead V2.

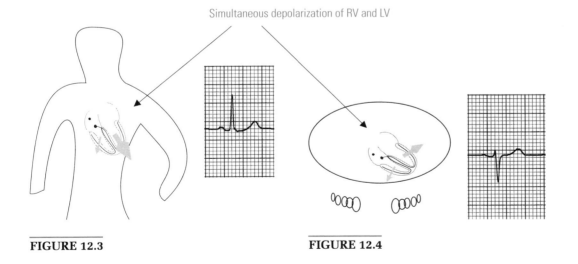

Simultaneous depolarization of RV and LV

FIGURE 12.3   **FIGURE 12.4**

Left Bundle Branch Block: Pathophysiology

In left bundle branch block (Figure 12.5), this all changes. The ventricles are not depolarized at the same time, but in sequence—first the right ventricle, then the left. The sequence begins with the right bundle, since it is functioning normally. It depolarizes the whole right ventricle in the normal amount of time, which is less than 0.08 seconds. The rest of the QRS after that first 0.08 seconds represents only left ventricular activation. This is the second part of the sequence, depolarization of the left ventricle from the efforts of the right bundle. Since the depolarization of both ventricles is not simultaneous but sequential, it takes 50% longer to finish compared with the normal QRS of 0.08 seconds. Prolongation of the QRS interval to 0.12 seconds or more is the diagnostic signature of bundle branch block. This sequential depolarization allows for the second hallmark of LBBB, namely, that the last part of the depolarization sequence (the QRS) must be left ventricular in direction. In LBBB, ventricular activation ends late and on the left side, so the QRS ends in the left ventricle, a direction that is toward the patient's left side and posterior.

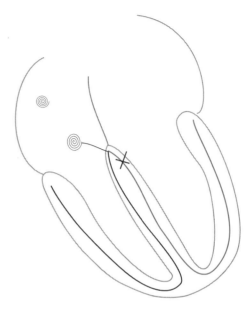

FIGURE 12.5

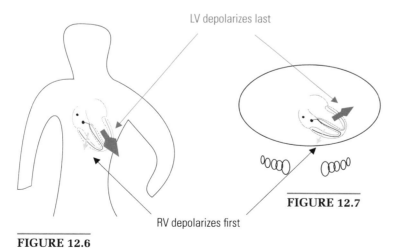

LV depolarizes last

RV depolarizes first

FIGURE 12.6

FIGURE 12.7

Left Bundle Branch Block: EKG in the Frontal Plane

Prolongation of the QRS interval to 0.12 seconds or more is the diagnostic signature of bundle branch block. **This sequential depolarization allows for the second hallmark of LBBB, namely, that the last part of the depolarization sequence (the QRS) must be left ventricular in direction.** In LBBB, ventricular activation ends late and on the left side, so the QRS ends in the left ventricle, a direction that is toward the patient's left side and posterior. **When the QRS interval is 0.12 seconds or more, bundle branch block is present.** Visualize the direction of the end of the QRS. If it points to the left ventricle, then LBBB is present. In the frontal plane view (Figure 12.8a), the last part of the sequence emanates from the left ventricle and points to the patient's left. Visualize the direction of the end of the QRS in lead I. Since it is positive, it points toward the left.

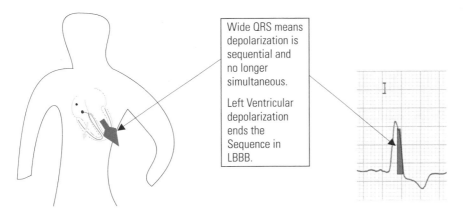

Wide QRS means depolarization is sequential and no longer simultaneous.

Left Ventricular depolarization ends the Sequence in LBBB.

FIGURE 12.8

Left Bundle Branch Block: EKG Findings in the Horizontal Plane

Prolongation of the QRS interval to 0.12 seconds or more is the diagnostic signature of bundle branch block. This sequential depolarization allows for the second hallmark of LBBB, namely that the last part of the depolarization sequence (the QRS) must be left ventricular in direction. **In LBBB, the right bundle finishes off ventricular activation on the left side, so the QRS ends in the left ventricle, a direction that is toward the patient's left side and posterior. When the QRS interval is 0.12 seconds or more, bundle branch block is present.** Visualize the direction of the end of the QRS in the horizontal plane. If it points to the left ventricle, then LBBB is present.

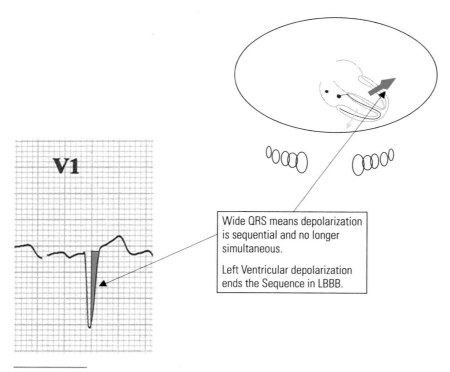

Wide QRS means depolarization is sequential and no longer simultaneous.

Left Ventricular depolarization ends the Sequence in LBBB.

FIGURE 12.9

Left Bundle Branch Block: Summary of Criteria

Criteria 1: The QRS interval is 0.12 seconds or longer

Criteria 2: The last part of the QRS is moving toward the left ventricle, which is left and posterior.

A) Limb Leads: The QRS ends in a positive wave (R or R′) in Lead I, and in V6. This is a leftward direction.

B) Horizontal Leads: The QRS ends in a negative (Q or QS) wave in Lead V1. This is a posterior and leftward direction

Critical Point: The first half of the QRS is irrelevant in making the diagnosis of LBBB!

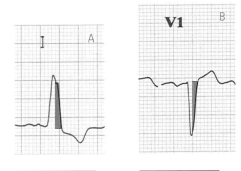

FIGURE 12.10   **FIGURE 12.11**

1

Left Bundle Branch Block

This is an example of LBBB. It meets the two criteria for diagnosis. First, the QRS interval is 0.12 seconds or more. This means the ventricles were not depolarized simultaneously, but sequentially. Since the ventricles are out of sequence, inspection of the last half of the QRS identifies the late or delayed ventricle. In Figure 12.12, the end of the QRS is positive in lead I (an R wave), and so points to the patient's left. The end of the QRS in lead V1 is negative, and so points posteriorly and leftward. In both leads I and V1, the delayed part of the QRS points to the left ventricle. Since the left ventricle is delayed, it must be the left bundle that is blocked.

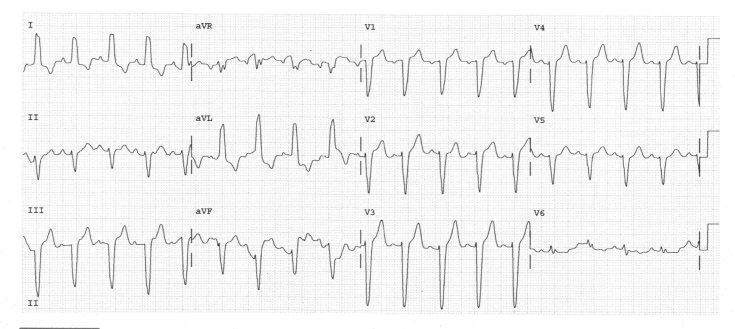

FIGURE 12.12

Left Bundle Branch Block:
Abnormal ST Segments

In LBBB, the ST segment is predictably abnormal and points away from the left ventricle. In Figure 12.13, the last part of the QRS is positive in lead I, so the ST segment should point away from this, or manifest ST segment depression in that lead. In lead V1 (Figure 12.14), the last part of the QRS is negative, so the ST segment should point away from that, or manifest ST segment elevation. In LBBB, the formation of the QRS is so abnormal that none of the criteria for analyzing the QRS, ST segment or T wave are particularly useful. Therefore, in LBBB, do not describe any further abnormalities! When LBBB is present, stop further EKG analysis. Do not diagnose hemiblock, infarction, ischemia, or hypertrophy.

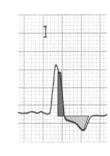

In Left Bundle Branch Block, expect the ST segment to point in the opposite direction from the last part of the QRS.

FIGURE 12.13

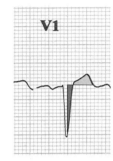

FIGURE 12.14

Left Bundle Branch Block:
Clinical Associations

There are five common classes of clinical associations in LBBB.
1) Coronary artery disease
2) Pressure overload
    a. Hypertension
    b. Aortic stenosis
    c. Hypertrophic cardiomyopathy
3) Volume overload
    a. Mitral regurgitation
    b. Aortic regurgitation
4) Dilated cardiomyopathy
5) Primary disease of the conduction system

Mechanical Contraction with a Normal QRS

To visualize ventricular contraction with a normal QRS, it is easier to view a cross-section of the heart. Figure 12.15 demonstrates a four-chamber view of the heart. A line through the middle of this view produces Figure 12.16. This cross-sectional view is usually called a short axis view. You can easily recognize it because the LV looks like a donut, or car tire. In a functioning ventricle with normal conduction, each of the four walls of the left ventricle (septum, anterior wall, lateral wall, and posterior wall) contracts normally and in synchronization toward the center of the left ventricular cavity. (In mechanical terms, the septum functions as an equal partner for the LV, not the RV.) This provides for normal cardiac systolic and diastolic function. In Figure 12.17, the patient has a severely dilated and hypokinetic left ventricle. Since the ventricle is so weak, it is very important for the four walls to contract in unison, however weak they are. With a normal QRS, the four walls of the left ventricle contract (however weakly) in the same direction, at the same time, and simultaneously with the right ventricle.

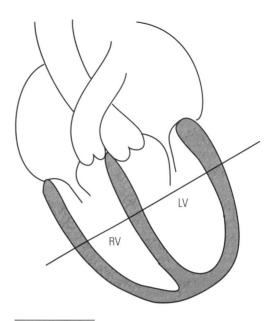

FIGURE 12.15

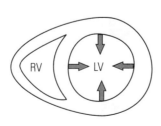

FIGURE 12.16

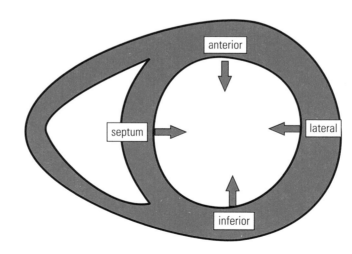

FIGURE 12.17

Left Bundle Branch Block: Cardiac Desynchronization

When the ventricles lose coordination in either direction or timing of contraction between parts of the left ventricle or between the left and right ventricles, desynchronization is present. Desynchronization hurts overall cardiac function and can worsen symptoms of systolic and diastolic heart failure. Figure 12.18 demonstrates a dilated cardiomyopathy. There are three ways that LBBB can hurt overall cardiac function in a patient with severe left ventricle dysfunction, as shown in Figure 12.19. First, the septum is depolarized by the right bundle, and so contracts the wrong way, namely toward the RV. This means one of the four weak walls (the septum) is not only not helping, but is going the wrong way and subtracting from the other walls' efforts. This is called a dyskinetic septum and can be diagnosed easily on echocardiography. Second, the delay between the activation of the septum and the far away left ventricular lateral wall is prolonged by at least 50%. Thus, the lateral wall and septum do not contract simultaneously, but sequentially. This significantly reduces whatever mechanical effectiveness the weak left ventricle has remaining. Third, the right ventricle depolarized normally and earlier, so blood is on the way from the right to the left ventricle before the left side is ready. The only place to put that blood is in the lungs, which leads to increased pulmonary congestion.

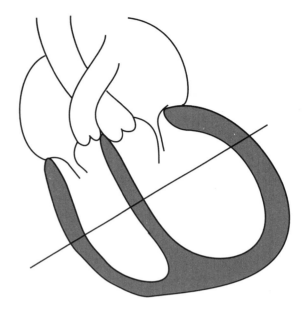

FIGURE 12.18

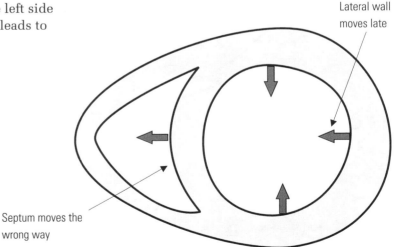

Lateral wall moves late

Septum moves the wrong way

FIGURE 12.19

Left Bundle Branch Block: How Resynchronization Therapy Works

Resynchronization therapy is used in situations where both severe left ventricular systolic function and bundle branch block are present. Two pacing leads are used for the left ventricle. One is placed inside the right ventricle at the apex (A). The second is placed either in the coronary sinus or on the outside surface of the lateral wall of the left ventricle (B). This dual pacing (biventricular pacing) effect provides simultaneous depolarization of the left ventricle from two different sides and helps to provide a more synchronized effort for the weakened walls.

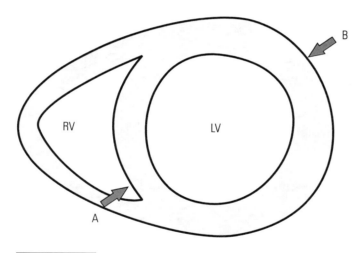

FIGURE 12.20

Incomplete Left Bundle Branch: Pathophysiology

Less than total loss of function in either the right or left bundle is called intra-ventricular conduction delay (IVCD) or incomplete LBBB. The primary diagnostic EKG abnormality in IVCD is prolongation of the QRS interval to 0.10 or 0.11 seconds. As in bundle branch block, IVCD may be left, right, or indeterminate. Once the QRS interval is measured at 0.10 or 0.11 seconds, it is the end of the QRS that is the key to diagnosis. If the end of the QRS is leftward (postive in lead I) and toward the left ventricle (negative in lead V1), then LIVCD is present.

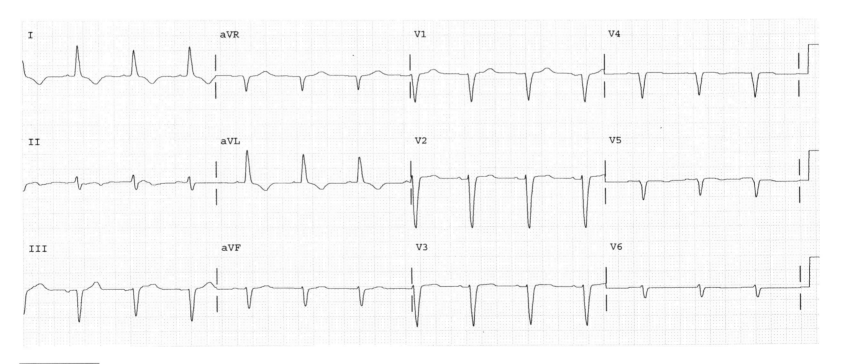

FIGURE 12.21

SAMPLE COMPLETED WORKSHEET

BASIC MEASUREMENTS

Parameter	Measurement	Interpretation
HR	86	Normal
Rhythm	Sinus	Normal
PR	0.16	Normal
QRS	0.14	LBBB
QT	0.38	
QTc	0.46	Long
P direction	Inferior and leftward	Normal
QRS direction		Not measured in LBBB

Instructions for Chapter 12 Worksheets

A) Complete basic measurements.
B) If the QRS is ≥ 0.12 sec, diagnose BBB. Then visualize the extra piece at the end of the QRS in the frontal plane as right or left, and in the horizontal plane as anterior or posterior. Diagnose BBB further as LBBB if the end of the QRS points to the left ventricle (leftward and posteriorly). Do not analyze the QRS, ST segment or T waves in LBBB. There are no agreed upon and reliable criteria for diagnosing ventricular hypertrophy, ischemia, or infarction in its presence.
C) Provide an interpretation.

Clinically Based Critical Thinking: Interpretation

LBBB is a very important finding on an EKG for two reasons. First (and unlike RBBB!) it is associated with underlying heart diease. Common associations with LBBB include coronary disease, hypertension, and cardiomyopathy. The cause of LBBB should be determined. Furthermore, the presence of systolic and disatolic dysfunction should be evaluated. Second, in LBBB (and unlike RBBB), the EKG cannot be further analyzed.

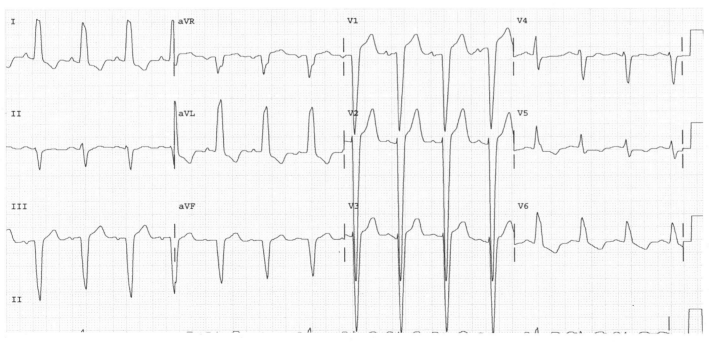

BASIC MEASUREMENTS

Parameter	Measurement	Interpretation
HR		
Rhythm		
PR		
QRS		
QT		
QTc		
P direction		
QRS direction		

Instructions for Chapter 12 Worksheets

A) Complete basic measurements.
B) If the QRS is ≥ 0.12 sec, diagnose BBB. Then visualize the extra piece at the end of the QRS in the frontal plane as right or left, and in the horizontal plane as anterior or posterior. Diagnose BBB further as LBBB if the end of the QRS points to the left ventricle (leftward and posteriorly). Do not analyze the QRS, ST segment or T waves in LBBB. There are no agreed upon and reliable criteria for diagnosing ventricular hypertrophy, ischemia, or infarction in its presence.
C) Provide an interpretation.

Clinically Based Critical Thinking: Interpretation

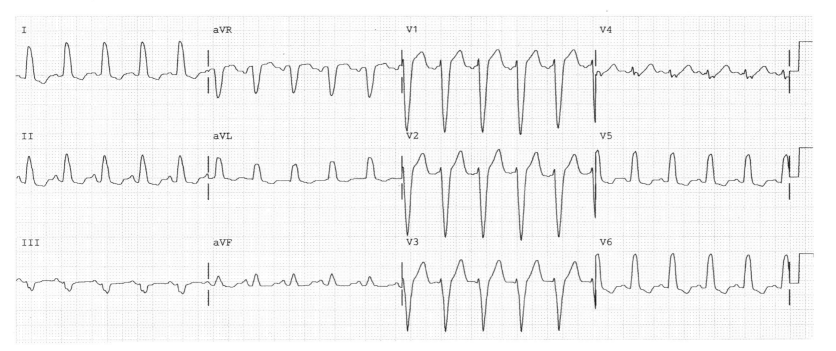

WORKSHEET 12.2

BASIC MEASUREMENTS		
Parameter	Measurement	Interpretation
HR		
Rhythm		
PR		
QRS		
QT		
QTc		
P direction		
QRS direction		

Instructions for Chapter 12 Worksheets

A) Complete basic measurements.
B) If the QRS is ≥ 0.12 sec, diagnose BBB. Then visualize the extra piece at the end of the QRS in the frontal plane as right or left, and in the horizontal plane as anterior or posterior. Diagnose BBB further as LBBB if the end of the QRS points to the left ventricle (leftward and posteriorly). Do not analyze the QRS, ST segment or T waves in LBBB. There are no agreed upon and reliable criteria for diagnosing ventricular hypertrophy, ischemia, or infarction in its presence.
C) Provide an interpretation.

Clinically Based Critical Thinking: Interpretation

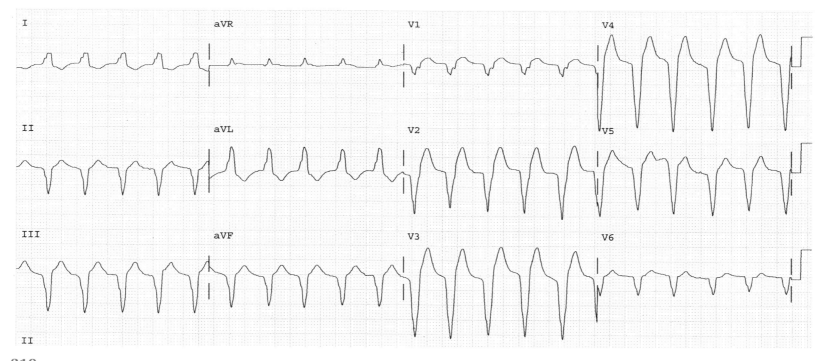

BASIC MEASUREMENTS		
Parameter	Measurement	Interpretation
HR		
Rhythm		
PR		
QRS		
QT		
QTc		
P direction		
QRS direction		

Instructions for Chapter 12 Worksheets

A) Complete basic measurements.
B) If the QRS is ≥ 0.12 sec, diagnose BBB. Then visualize the extra piece at the end of the QRS in the frontal plane as right or left, and in the horizontal plane as anterior or posterior. Diagnose BBB further as LBBB if the end of the QRS points to the left ventricle (leftward and posteriorly). Do not analyze the QRS, ST segment or T waves in LBBB. There are no agreed upon and reliable criteria for diagnosing ventricular hypertrophy, ischemia, or infarction in its presence.
C) Provide an interpretation.

Clinically Based Critical Thinking: Interpretation

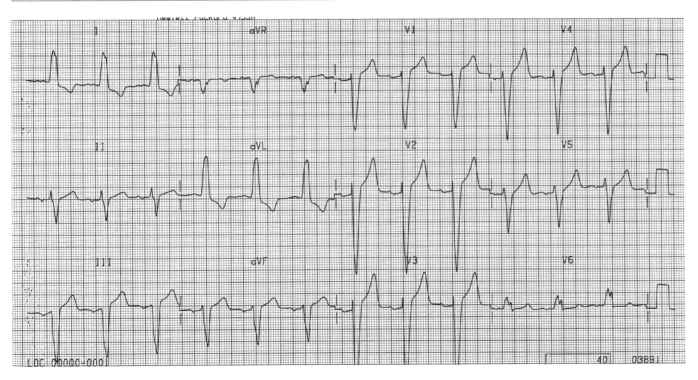

WORKSHEET IV.1

Clinically Based Critical Thinking: Interpretation

BASIC MEASUREMENTS		
Parameter	**Measurement**	**Interpretation**
HR		
Rhythm		
PR		
QRS		
QT		
QTc		
P direction		
QRS direction		

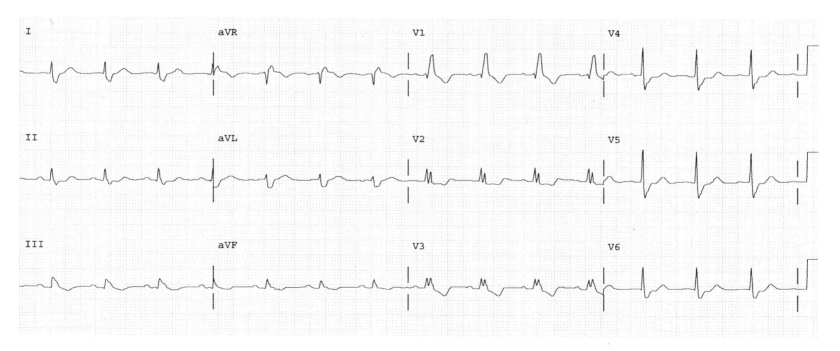

Clinically Based Critical Thinking: Interpretation

BASIC MEASUREMENTS		
Parameter	Measurement	Interpretation
HR		
Rhythm		
PR		
QRS		
QT		
QTc		
P direction		
QRS direction		

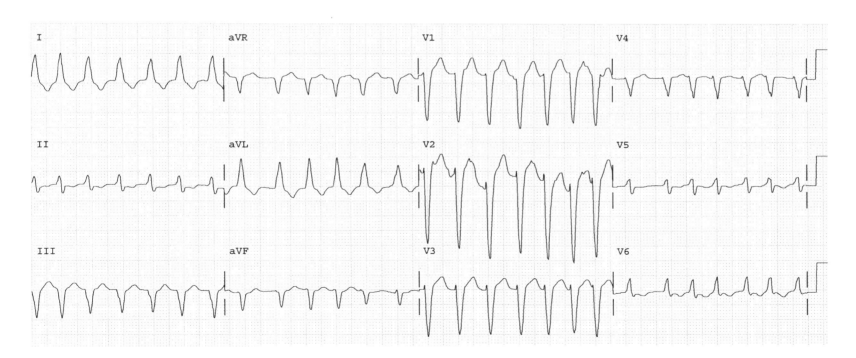

Clinically Based Critical Thinking: Interpretation

BASIC MEASUREMENTS		
Parameter	Measurement	Interpretation
HR		
Rhythm		
PR		
QRS		
QT		
QTc		
P direction		
QRS direction		

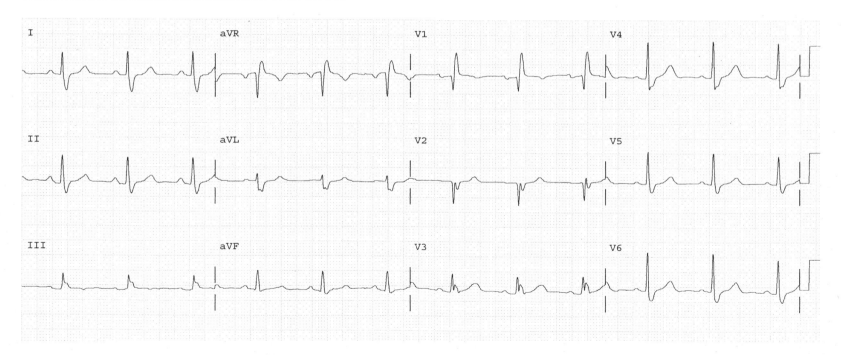

WORKSHEET IV.4

BASIC MEASUREMENTS		
Parameter	Measurement	Interpretation
HR		
Rhythm		
PR		
QRS		
QT		
QTc		
P direction		
QRS direction		

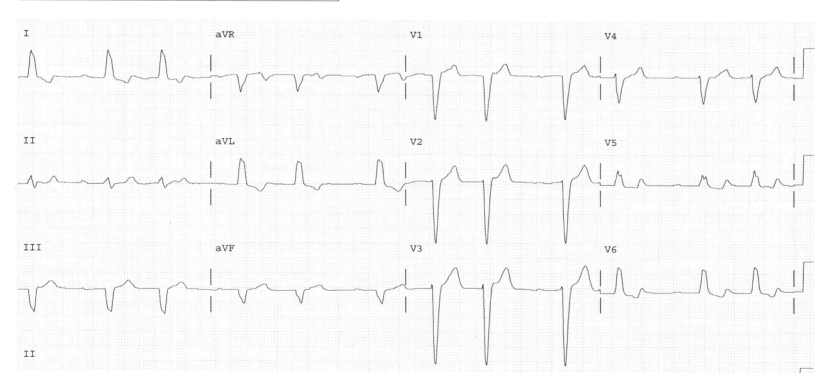

WORKSHEET IV.5

BASIC MEASUREMENTS

Parameter	Measurement	Interpretation
HR		
Rhythm		
PR		
QRS		
QT		
QTc		
P direction		
QRS direction		

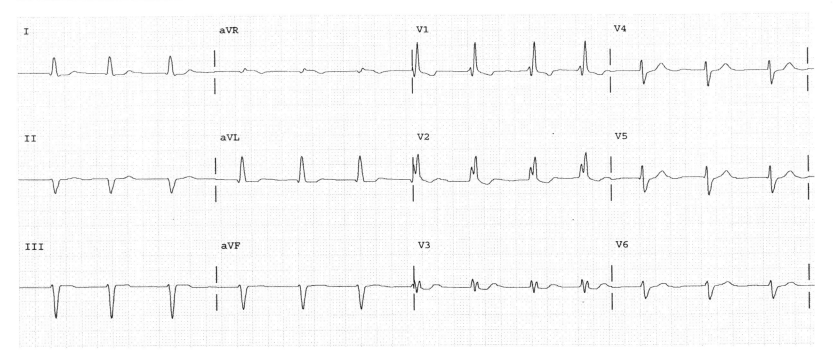

The Ischemic Disorders: EKG Changes Related to Ischemia and Myocardial Infarction (MI)

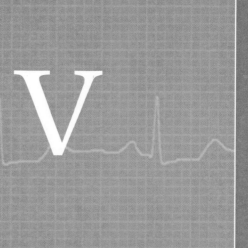

The Partially-Occluded Artery: Angina and Non-ST Elevation MI

The Normal T Wave

The T wave is normally the last complex in the cardiac cycle. It represents electrical activity produced during rapid ventricular repolarization. The repolarization process allows the depolarized cardiac cells to reset for the next cardiac cycle, much like a rubber band has to be restretched before it can be released. Repolarization requires a constant supply of oxygen rich blood flow to supply energy for this process. The direction of the normal repolarization wave is similar to that of the depolarization wave. We can visualize the direction of the normal T wave axis as pointing inferiorly and to the patient's left, which is toward the apex of left ventricle, much as the QRS does (Figures 13.1, 13.2).

Self-Study Objectives

- **Define and identify the following:**

  Normal T wave

  Direction of T wave changes in ischemia

  Location of ischemia in the myocardium

- **List two clinical mechanisms of worsening ischemia**

- **List two clinical mechanisms of ameliorating ischemia**

- **Describe the coronary arteries and the structures they supply**

- **Describe the pathophysiology of stable angina**

- **Describe the pathophysiology of the acute coronary syndrome**

- **Name the three rules of the T waves**

- **Describe the inverted T wave patterns for localizing ischemia and infarction**

- **Describe the significance of ST segment depression**

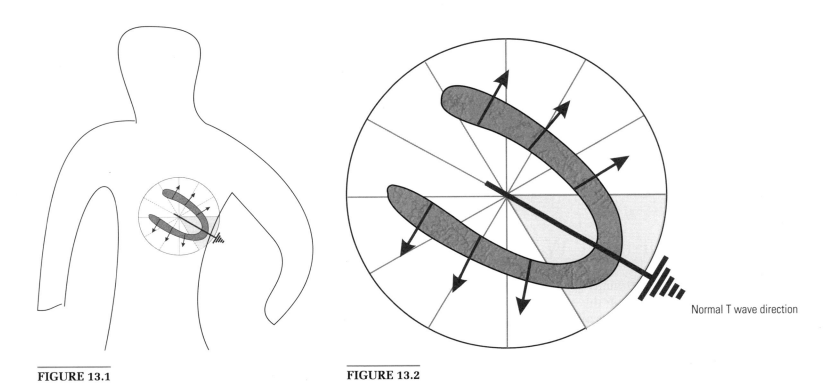

FIGURE 13.1

FIGURE 13.2

Normal T wave direction

The T Wave in Ischemia: Overview

The T wave represents electrical activity produced during the rapid ventricular repolarization. This active process of repolarization requires a constant supply of oxygen to generate energy. If too little oxygenated blood flow is available for the metabolic needs of the tissues, ischemia results. Ischemic areas cannot generate energy to repolarize as readily as nonischemic cells, so the direction of repolarization changes. On the EKG, this appears as a T wave direction pointing away from an area of ischemia. Drug effects and electrolyte abnormalities are also important causes of T wave changes, as is discussed in Chapter 19.

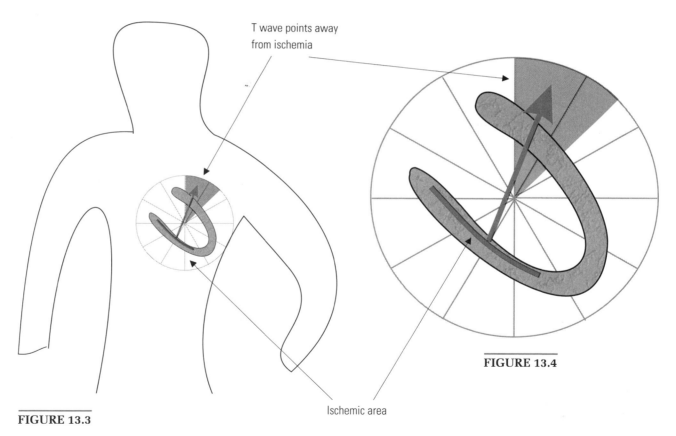

T wave points away from ischemia

Ischemic area

FIGURE 13.4

FIGURE 13.3

Location of Ischemia: The Vulnerable Subendocardium

The part of the myocardium most distant from the arteries is the subendocardial region. The subendocardium is the furthest away from the arteries, which must penetrate through contracting muscle to deliver the blood to the subendocardial layer. This makes the subendocardial region the most sensitive to ischemic conditions, such as increased demand or decreased supply. Any increase in demand or decrease in supply of blood at the level of the subendocardium can produce ischemia. If the ischemic conditions are severe, not soon relieved, or both, then infarction (cell death) occurs.

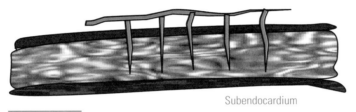

Subendocardium

FIGURE 13.5

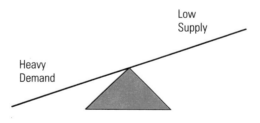

Low Supply

Heavy Demand

FIGURE 13.6

Clinical Mechanisms of Ischemia

Ischemia occurs when there is an imbalance between the supply of oxygen to the myocardium and the demand for oxygen by the myocardial mitochondria. Any increase in demand or decrease in supply may cause ischemia and, if it continues, can lead to tissue infarction. The effects of these precipitating causes are additive.

Oxygen demand is increased by:

1. Tachycardia
2. Increased blood pressure
3. Increased heart size (harder to squeeze a basketball than a grape).

Oxygen supply is decreased by

1. Low hemoglobin
2. Low pO_2
3. Fixed atherosclerotic narrowing
4. A growing atherosclerotic obstruction
5. Coronary artery spasm

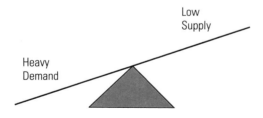

FIGURE 13.7

Clinical Mechanisms That Can Relieve Ischemia

Ischemia occurs when there is an imbalance between the supply of oxygen to the myocardium and the demand for oxygen by the myocardial mitochondria. Therapeutic goals in this setting are to either increase the supply, decrease the demand, or both.

Any decrease in demand or increase in supply may help relieve ischemia. If the therapeutic intervention is done effectively and quickly, it can prevent the progression to permanent cell death (infarction) of myocardial tissue. If the interventions are not successful, myocardial infarction occurs.

Oxygen demand is decreased by:

1. Decreasing a high heart rate
2. Decreasing a high blood pressure
3. Decreasing a dilated heart size

Oxygen supply is increased by

1. Increasing a low hemoglobin
2. Increasing a low pO_2
3. Dilating or bypassing a fixed lesion
4. Decreasing coronary artery spasm, if present

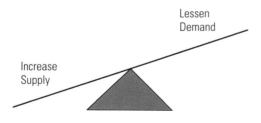

FIGURE 13.8

Anatomy and Pathophysiology of Ischemia: Stable Angina

The heart normally receives fully oxygenated blood through the right and left coronary arteries. The process of conduction and contraction is energy dependent on a second-to-second basis, and a lack of blood flow can cause problems quickly. Atherosclerotic plaque is the most common underlying cause that creates blockages in these arteries, thereby reducing the supply of oxygen to the ventricle. The obstructive process can occur slowly over years and, at the beginning (Figure 13.9), may not cause any symptoms. As the cross-sectional area of the epicardial artery decreases (Figure 13.10), the supply of blood also decreases. This fixed obstruction causes the classic exertionally provoked, rest-relieved symptoms of stable angina.

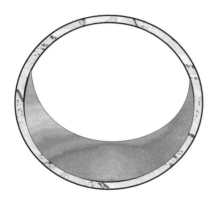

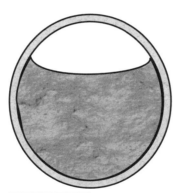

FIGURE 13.10

FIGURE 13.9

Pathophysiology of Ischemia: Acute Coronary Syndrome

The process of atherosclereosis can occur slowly over years. At the beginning (as shown in Figure 13.9), it may not cause any symptoms. This can change in a matter of minutes. An atherosclerotic plaque can unpredictably and acutely rupture and spill its fatty contents (Figure 13.11) into the arterial lumen. This plaque rupture can immediately cause a thrombus to form on top of the partial blockage from the underlying plaque (Figure 13.12) and produce a sudden change in the patient's symptoms. This is called an acute coronary syndrome.

Regardless of the mechanism causing the obstruction (the one-component large plaque of stable angina or the two-component plaque-with-thrombus of acute coronary syndrome), the area of the ventricle with poor blood supply has less oxygen than it needs. Less oxygen translates immediately into less energy. This interferes with the ischemic area's ability to repolarize normally, and we see this as a directional change in the T wave.

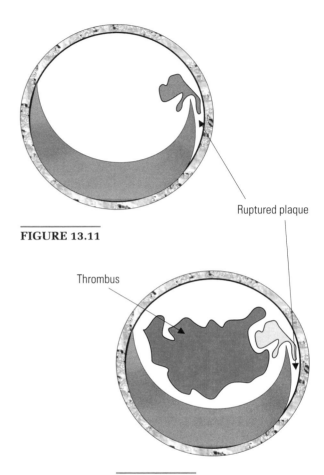

FIGURE 13.11

Ruptured plaque

Thrombus

FIGURE 13.12

The First Rule of the T Waves

Any process that causes ischemia can eventually result in infarction (cell death) if it is prolonged or severe enough. Ischemia, by interfering with normal repolarization, changes the direction of the T wave away from the ischemic area. If infarction occurs, the T wave may remain permanently abnormal. This creates a common problem for an EKG reader that can be summed up as The First Rule of the T Waves. It states: On a single EKG-in-hand, neither ST depression nor T wave changes can prove timing or reversibility. This simply stated rule is probably the least understood principle in all of electrocardiography. If a pattern of T wave inversion or ST depression is present (see Table 13.1), it makes the presence of significant obstructive coronary disease likely. It does not distinguish whether the event is new or old. Furthermore, if the finding of T wave inversion or ST depression is found to be new, it still does not determine (on that single EKG!) whether the process is reversible or permanent. If the T or ST abnormalities are unchanged compared to an old EKG, they represent an old and irreversible process, a non-ST elevation MI. If the changes are new compared to an old EKG, they represent an acute coronary syndrome—unstable angina or a new non-ST elevation MI. To separate these three possibilities, we need additional information. The old EKG is helpful in deciding whether or not the EKG changes are new. A follow-up EKG is helpful in deciding if the EKG changes are reversible.

TABLE 13.1

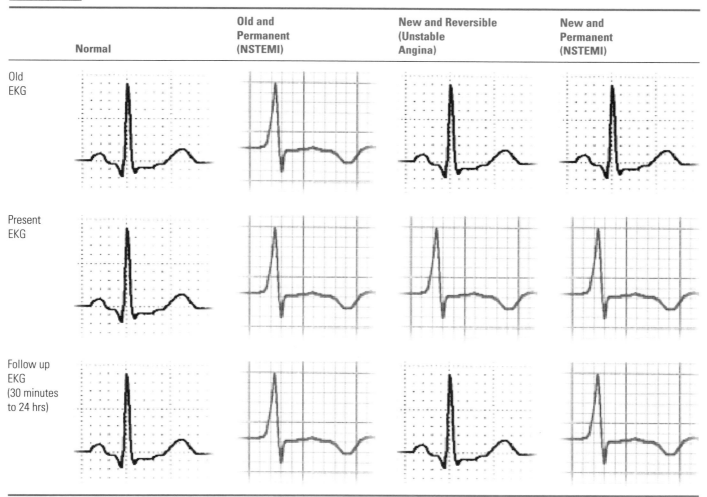

	Normal	Old and Permanent (NSTEMI)	New and Reversible (Unstable Angina)	New and Permanent (NSTEMI)
Old EKG				
Present EKG				
Follow up EKG (30 minutes to 24 hrs)				

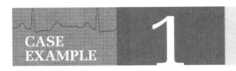

1

Inferior Ischemia or Infarction

EKG: The T wave is negative in leads II, III, and AVF, but positive in I and AVL (Figure 3.13).

Visualization: The T is pointing to the left and superiorly, away from the inferior wall (Figure 3.14).

Critical Thinking: The T wave is pointing away from the inferior wall. The right coronary artery (RCA) supplies blood to the inferior and posterior walls. We expect a significant obstruction with either a plaque (or a plaque plus a clot) in that artery. Since we have no other information and only a single EKG, the First Rule of the T Waves applies (Figure 13.21). This provides a differential diagnosis of three likely possibilities. First, these T waves could be old, unchanged from a previous non-ST elevation MI. Second, these T waves could be new and changed from a previously normal EKG, but may reverse in the next (in 30 minutes or several hours) EKG. This would indicate a new reversible ischemic process called unstable angina. Third, these T waves could be new but not reverse within 24 hours. They would then typically be associated with a positive blood test of biochemical markers such as Troponin. This would confirm an irreversible loss of myocardial cells called non-ST elevation myocardial infarction (NSTEMI).

Pattern to Memorize: The T waves point away (−45° to −90°) from leads II, III and AVF, giving an inverted T wave in these leads.

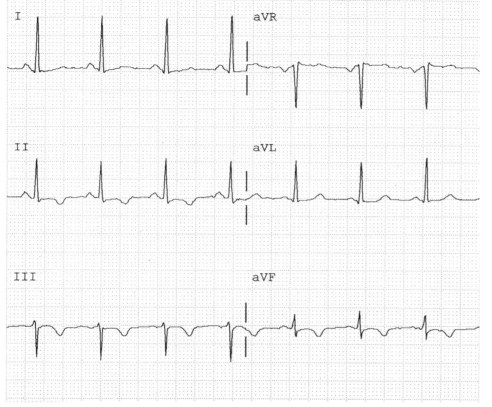

FIGURE 13.13

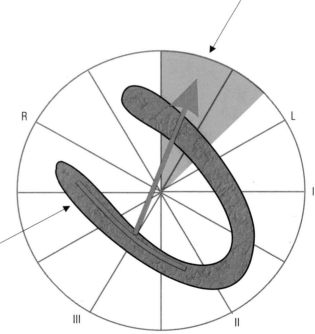

T wave points away from ischemic or infarcted interior wall

Interior wall is ischemic or infarcted

FIGURE 13.14

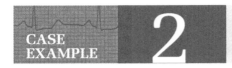

CASE EXAMPLE 2 — Lateral Wall Ischemia or Infarction

EKG: The T wave is negative in leads I and AVL, but positive in III and AVF.

Visualization: The T is pointing to the patient's right side, away from the lateral wall (Figure 13.16).

Critical Thinking: Since the T wave is pointing away from the lateral wall, we locate the area of ischemia or infarction here. The left coronary artery supplies blood to the anterior and lateral walls. We expect a significant obstruction with either a plaque (or a plaque plus a clot) in the LAD or circumflex artery. Again, if we have no other information, we apply the First Rule of the T Waves. This provides a differential diagnosis of three likely possibilities (Figure 13.21). First, these T waves could be old, unchanged from a previous non-ST elevation MI. Second, these T waves could be new and changed from a previously normal EKG, but may reverse in the next (in 30 minutes or several hours) EKG. This would indicate a new reversible ischemic process called unstable angina. Third, these T waves could be new but not reverse within 24 hours. They would then typically be associated with a positive blood test of biochemical markers such as Troponin. This would confirm an irreversible loss of myocardial cells called non-ST elevation myocardial infarction (NSTEMI).

Pattern to Memorize: The T waves point away (+105° to +180°) from leads I and AVL, giving an inverted T wave in these leads.

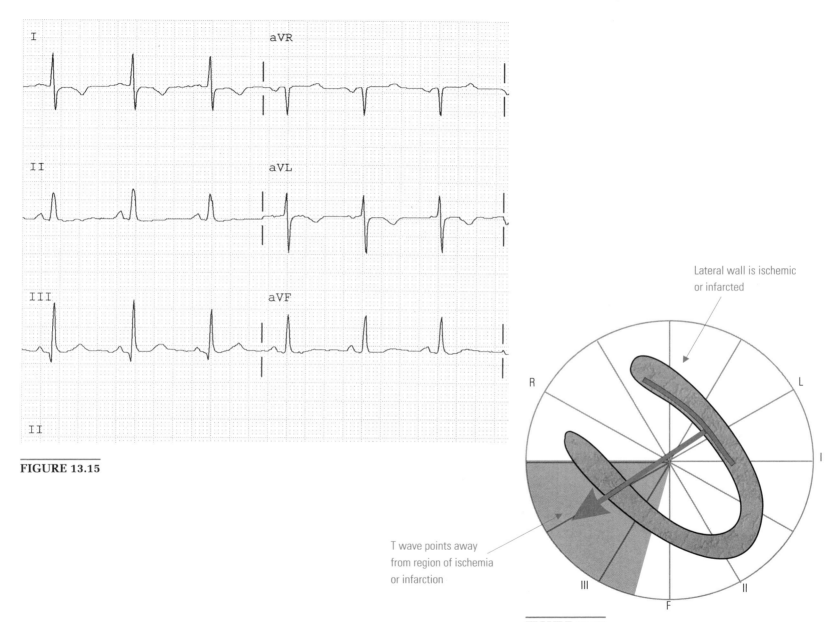

FIGURE 13.15

Lateral wall is ischemic or infarcted

T wave points away from region of ischemia or infarction

FIGURE 13.16

Apical Ischemia or Infarction

EKG: The T wave is negative in leads I and AVF (Figure 13.17).

Visualization: The T is pointing superiorly and to the patient's right side, away from the apex (Figure 13.18).

Critical Thinking: Since the T wave is pointing away from the apex, we locate the area of ischemia or infarction here. The left coronary artery supplies blood to the apex. We expect a significant obstruction with either a plaque (or a plaque plus a clot) in the LAD. Again, if we have no other information, we apply the First Rule of the T Waves. This provides a differential diagnosis of three likely possibilities. First, these T waves could be old, unchanged from a previous non-ST elevation MI. Second, these T waves could be new and changed from a previously normal EKG, but may reverse in the next (in 30 minutes or several hours) EKG. This would indicate a new reversible ischemic process called unstable angina. Third, these T waves could be new but not reverse within 24 hours. They would then typically be associated with a positive blood test of biochemical markers such as Troponin. This would confirm an irreversible loss of myocardial cells called non-ST elevation myocardial infarction (NSTEMI).

Pattern to Memorize: The T waves point away (−105° to −165°) from leads I and AVF, giving an inverted T wave in these leads.

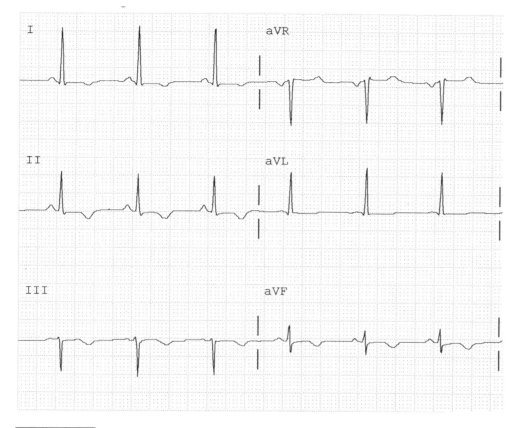

FIGURE 13.17

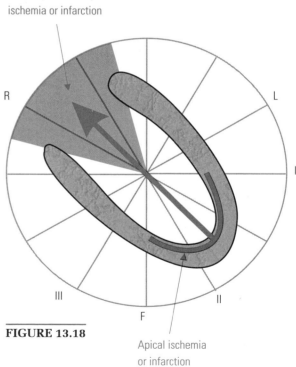

T wave points away from ischemia or infarction

R

L

I

III

II

F

FIGURE 13.18

Apical ischemia or infarction

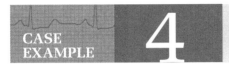

Septal and Anterior Ischemia or Infarction

EKG: The T wave is negative in leads V1, V2, V3, and V4 (Figure 13.19).

Visualization: The T is pointing posteriorly, away from the septum and anterior walls (Figure 13.20).

Critical Thinking: Since the T wave is pointing away from the septum and anterior walls, we locate the area of ischemia or infarction here. The left coronary artery supplies blood to the septum and anterior walls. We expect a significant obstruction with either a plaque (or a plaque plus a clot) in the LAD. Again, if we have no other information, we apply the First Rule of the T Waves. This provides a differential diagnosis of three likely possibilities. First, these T waves could be old, unchanged from a previous non-ST elevation MI. Second, these T waves could be new and changed from a previously normal EKG, but may reverse in the next (in 30 minutes or several hours) EKG. This would indicate a new reversible ischemic process called unstable angina. Third, these T waves could be new but not reverse within 24 hours. They would then typically be associated with a positive blood test of biochemical markers such as Troponin. This would confirm an irreversible loss of myocardial cells called non-ST elevation myocardial infarction (NSTEMI).

Pattern to Memorize: The T waves point away (−22.5° to −60°) from leads V1, V2 and V3, giving an inverted T wave in these leads.

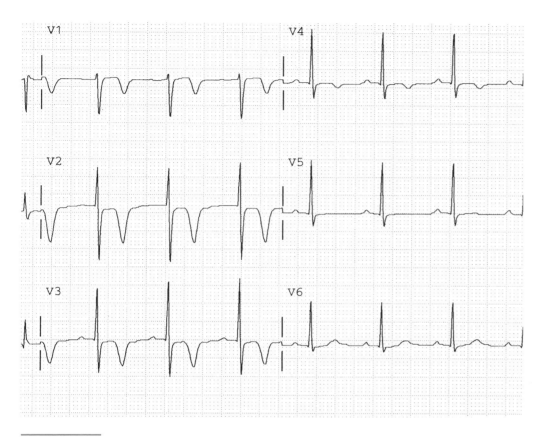

FIGURE 13.19

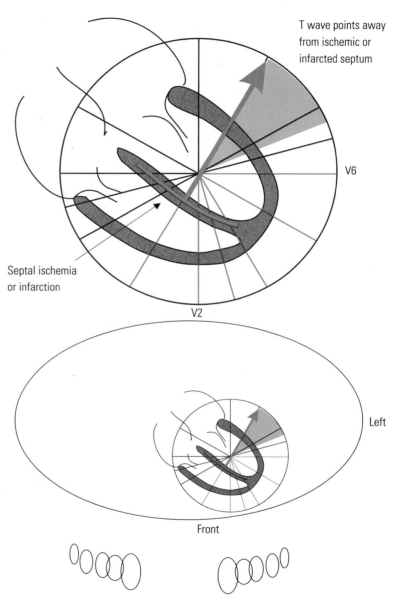

T wave points away from ischemic or infarcted septum

V6

Septal ischemia or infarction

V2

Left

Front

FIGURE 13.20

MEMORIZE THIS!   **Location of the T Wave: Frontal Plane Patterns**

Location of Process (Ischemia or NSTEMI)	Visualize the Concept	Memorize These Patterns
Inferior	T waves point away from inferior wall	II, III, AVF
Lateral	T waves point away from lateral wall	I, AVL
Apical	T waves point away from apex	I, AVF
Nonspecific inferior T wave changes	T waves borderline superior	III, AVF, but not II
Nonspecific lateral T wave changes	T waves borderline rightward	L, but not I
Normal T axis	T waves point toward the apex	If any, only III
Nonspecific septal T wave changes	T wave points borderline away from the septum	V1 only
Septal	T wave points away from septum	V1 and V2
Anterior	T wave points away from the anterior wall	V3 and V4
Lateral	T wave points away from the lateral wall	V5 and V6
Nonspecific lateral T wave changes	T wave points borderline away from the lateral	V6 only
Normal	T wave toward the apex	No T wave inversion

The ST Segment: The Second Rule of the T Wave

The ST segment represents electrical activity produced during ventricular re-polarization. Normally, the ST segment is at the baseline since only an even exchange of charges is taking place as ions inside and outside the cell change places to be ready for the next QRS. In severe subendocardial ischemia, the ST segment can become abnormal and point away from regions of subendo-cardial ischemia. It is a more specific finding of subendocardial ischemia than T wave inversion. The Second Rule of the T Waves states: On a single EKG, if T wave changes and ST depression are both present, the ST segment depres-sion is more significant. Consider ischemia as a process of overheating the myocardium. Smelling smoke would be comparable to seeing an inverted pattern of T waves. Seeing smoke would compare to the presence of ST seg-ment depression. ST depression is not only more specific than T wave inver-sion for an ischemic process, it also carries a worse prognosis. Consider T wave inversion as the cell running out of energy at the very end of the repolar-ization cycle, while ST depression is a severe lack of enough energy from the very start of repolarization. In addition, downsloping ST segment depression is more specific than horizontal ST segment depression. Both are more spe-cific than upsloping ST segment depression.

TABLE 13.2   T wave and ST Segment Clinical Summary

Abnormal Pattern of T Wave Inversion or ST Depression		
New compared with old EKG or patient has symptoms		Unchanged compared with old EKG and patient has no symptoms
Follow-up EKG normalizes and biochemical markers negative	Follow-up EKG remains abnormal after 24 hours or biochemical markers positive	Old NSTEMI
Unstable Angina	New NSTEMI	

SAMPLE COMPLETED WORKSHEET

BASIC MEASUREMENTS			EVALUATION FOR ISCHEMIA OR INFARCTION	
Parameter	Measurement	Interpretation	Abnormal Parameter	If present, note the leads (or location) that contain the abnormality
HR	100	Abnormal	Inverted T waves	
Rhythm	Sinus	Normal		
PR	.16	Normal	ST depression	Diffuse
QRS	.08	Normal		
QT	0.30			
QTc	0.39	Normal	ST Elevation	
P direction	Inferior and leftward	Normal	Q Waves or equivalents	
QRS direction		Normal		

Instructions for Chapter 13 Worksheets

A) Complete basic measurements.
B) Do all previous work.
C) Note if inverted T waves or ST segment depression is present in two or more leads that represent a pattern in Table 13.1. Here the ST segments are diffusely abnormal.
D) Provide an interpretation.

Clinically Based Critical Thinking: Interpretation

ST segment depression is consistent with ischemia or infarction. On a single EKG, the First Rule of the T wave applies. The ST depression may represent infarction, which may be new, or old. It may also represent ischemia. More information is needed. Is the patient symptomatic? Is there an old EKG available? If so, are these ST changes new?

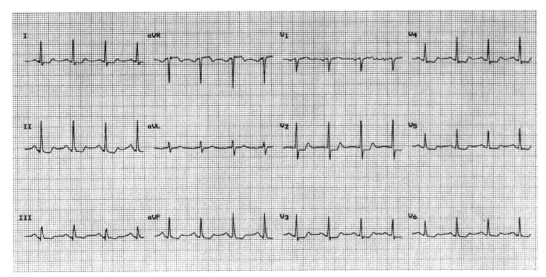

BASIC MEASUREMENTS			EVALUATION FOR ISCHEMIA OR INFARCTION	
Parameter	Measurement	Interpretation	Abnormal Parameter	If present, note the leads (or location) that contain the abnormality
HR			Inverted T waves	
Rhythm				
PR			ST depression	
QRS				
QT				
QTc			ST Elevation	
P direction			Q Waves or equivalents	
QRS direction				

Instructions for Chapter 13 Worksheets

A) Complete basic measurements.
B) Do all previous work.
C) Note if inverted T waves or ST segment depression is present in two or more leads that represent a pattern in Table 13.1.
D) Provide an interpretation.

Clinically Based Critical Thinking: Interpretation

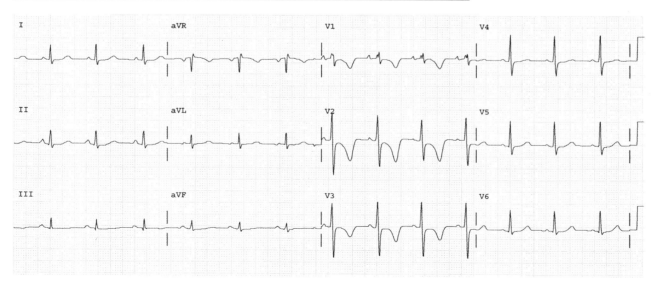

BASIC MEASUREMENTS			EVALUATION FOR ISCHEMIA OR INFARCTION	
Parameter	Measurement	Interpretation	Abnormal Parameter	If present, note the leads (or location) that contain the abnormality
HR			Inverted T waves	
Rhythm				
PR			ST depression	
QRS				
QT				
QTc			ST Elevation	
P direction			Q Waves or equivalents	
QRS direction				

Instructions for Chapter 13 Worksheets

A) Complete basic measurements.
B) Do all previous work.
C) Note if inverted T waves or ST segment depression is present in two or more leads that represent a pattern in Table13.1.
D) Provide an interpretation.

Clinically Based Critical Thinking: Interpretation

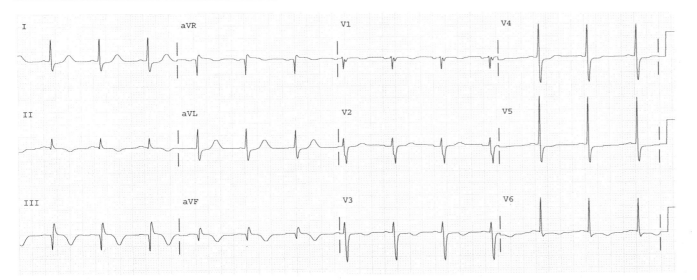

BASIC MEASUREMENTS			EVALUATION FOR ISCHEMIA OR INFARCTION	
Parameter	Measurement	Interpretation	Abnormal Parameter	If present, note the leads (or location) that contain the abnormality
HR			Inverted T waves	
Rhythm				
PR			ST depression	
QRS				
QT				
QTc			ST Elevation	
P direction			Q Waves or equivalents	
QRS direction				

Instructions for Chapter 13 Worksheets

A) Complete basic measurements.
B) Do all previous work.
C) Note if inverted T waves or ST segment depression is present in two or more leads that represent a pattern in Table 13.1.
D) Provide an interpretation.

Clinically Based Critical Thinking: Interpretation

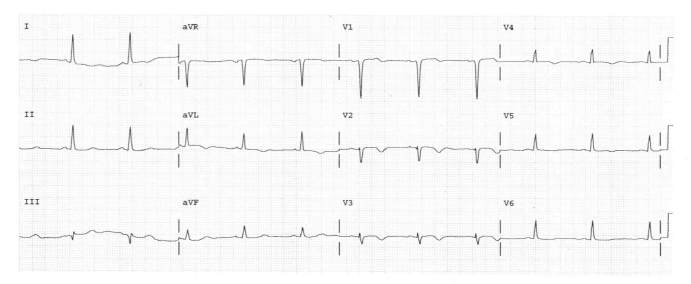

The Totally Occluded Artery: ST Elevation MI

14

ST Segment Elevation: An Overview

The ST segment represents electrical activity produced during ventricular repolarization. Normally, the ST segment is at the baseline because only an even exchange of charges is taking place, as ions inside and outside the cell exchange places to be ready for the next QRS. Ions normally move only through specialized ion doors (channels) in the otherwise impermeable cell membrane. These channels completely control the entry and exit of each ion. The ion channels require energy to function, and loss of energy production from ischemia affects the cell's ability to control overall ion flow, direction, and balance. Cell death from severe ischemia generates holes in the cells, and ions can flow freely in and out bypassing the channels completely. In addition to ischemia, inflammation, drugs, electrolyte abnormalities, and genetic variation can each affect the normal function of these cardiac channels. ST elevation can be seen in bundle branch block, hypertrophy, and pericarditis.

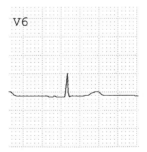

FIGURE 14.1

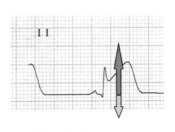

FIGURE 14.2

243

ST Elevation: Pathophysiology

ST segment elevation in two neighboring (contiguous) leads, in the setting of appropriate symptoms, typically represents a 100% blockage in a coronary artery. The occlusion has two components. The first is an underlying atherosclerotic plaque. This plaque accumulated slowly, over a period of years, on the inside wall of the coronary artery. At this point (Figure 14.3), the lesion may not have been large enough to obstruct blood flow either at rest or with stress. The patient may have had no previous symptoms, and a stress test would have been negative. This all changes with the development of an acute coronary syndrome. It begins with an unpredictable rupture of that atherosclerotic plaque, which pours highly thrombogenic material on top of the plaque (Figure 14.4). This immediately attracts and activates the coagulation system. A thrombus forms at the site of the ruptured plaque and forms the second component of the blockage (figure 14.5). When the thrombus combines with the underlying ruptured plaque, it can completely occlude 100% of the arterial lumen. This reduces the oxygen supply to zero producing extreme ischemia across a large layer of myocardium. This is called transmural ischemia, or ST segment elevation MI (STEMI). Although the terminology seems irreversible, immediate opening of the artery can salvage much of the myocardium. The disruption in ionic control produces the classic ST segment finding which is attracted to the part of the ventricle supplied by the blocked artery.

Thrombogenic material from ruptured plaque

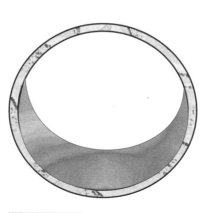

FIGURE 14.3

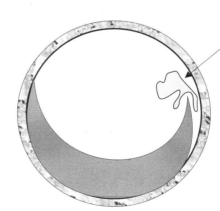

FIGURE 14.4

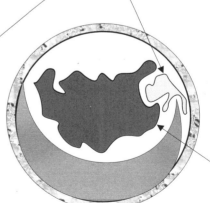

Occlusive thrombus

FIGURE 14.5

Location of Ischemia

Complete occlusion of a coronary artery represents the extreme case of supply and demand mismatch. **The region of ischemia involves not just the sub-endocardium, but the entire thickness of myocardium. Therefore, it is called "transmural" ischemia.** Clinically, it is called ST elevation MI (STEMI).

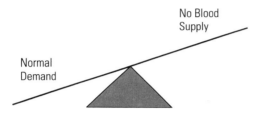

FIGURE 14.6

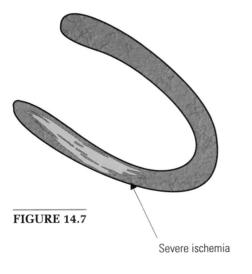

FIGURE 14.7

Severe ischemia

STEMI: The Third Rule of the T Waves

The third rule of T waves states: On a single EKG, if ST elevation is present in two contiguous leads, ignore the presence of T wave inversion and even ST depression. ST elevation is the primary process. In our previous analogy, overheating myocardium produced the smell of smoke (T wave inversion), or visible smoke (ST depression). ST elevation is seeing the myocardium in flames. There is no longer any question as to the next action. Diagnose Acute STEMI. Call the appropriate "Code MI" in your hospital. If you have a capable experienced interventional lab, notify the personnel immediately. The clock has started on rescuing the myocardium trapped without oxygen behind the 100% occlusion.

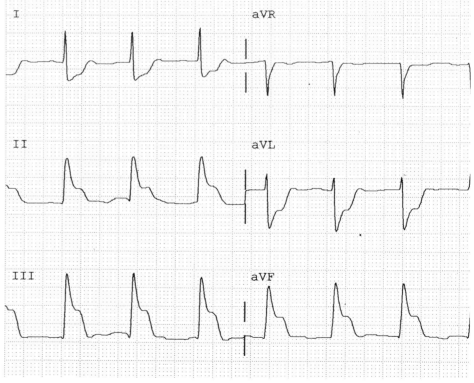

FIGURE 14.8

Treatment of STEMI: Primary Angioplasty vs. Thrombolysis

Immediate recognition of ST segment elevation on an EKG allows for surgical intervention to open the closed artery.

In the absence of an immediately available interventional lab, administration of thrombolytic drugs can dissolve the thrombus that overlies the ruptured atherosclerotic plaque. Intravenous thrombolytic therapy takes less time to administer than arranging for emergency angioplasty, but has a greater risk of severe hemorrhage. Figure 14.9a demonstrates an occlusion of the LAD artery, which opens up in Figure 14.9b after therapy.

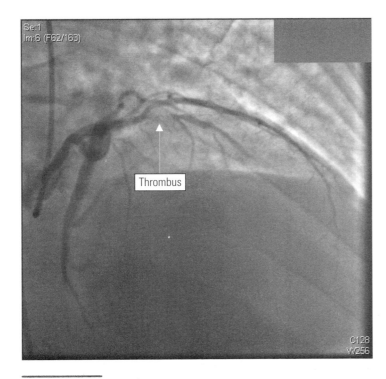

FIGURE 14.9a

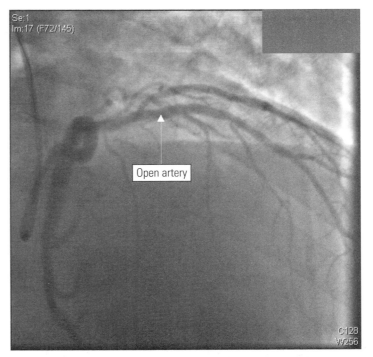

FIGURE 14.9b

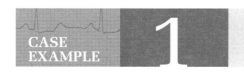

CASE
EXAMPLE

Inferior STEMI: Syndrome of RCA Occlusion

EKG: The ST segment is positive in leads III and AVF (Figure 14.10).

Visualization: The ST is pointing to the patient's right side, which is toward the inferior wall (Figure 14.11).

Critical Thinking: Since the ST segment is pointing toward the inferior wall (Figure 14.10), we locate the area of extreme or transmural ischemia here (Figure 14.11). The right coronary artery (RCA) supplies blood to the AV node and inferior wall through its posterior descending artery branch (PDA). We expect a significant obstruction with a ruptured plaque and a superimposed thombus in the RCA or PDA. We apply the Third Rule of the T Waves. We ignore the T wave changes and ST depression in leads I and AVl, and diagnose ST elevation myocardial infarction (NSTEMI). The right coronary artery supplies the right ventricle with blood. Right ventricular infarction may be present. Right ventricular infarction can cause right-sided heart failure and hypovolemic shock without pulmonary edema, since it is too weak to pump sufficient blood to the left ventricle. The RCA supplies the AV node 90% of the time, therefore heart block such as 1° AV block, Wenckebach, or complete heart block may be associated as well. A vagal response, with sinus bradycardia, nausea, and vomiting may also be associated. The posterior part of the ventricular septum may rarely rupture (producing an acquired ventricular septal defect) as a complication of RCA occlusion.

MEMORIZE THIS!

Pattern to Memorize

The ST waves point toward (+90° to +165°) leads III and AVF, producing ST elevation in these leads.

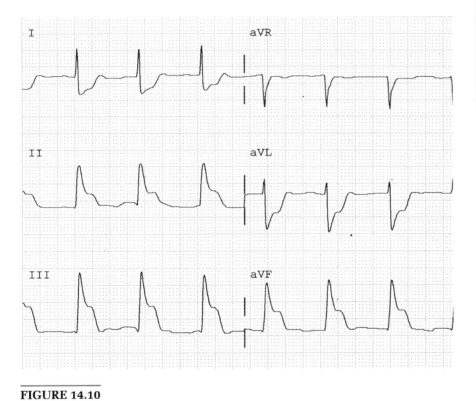

FIGURE 14.10

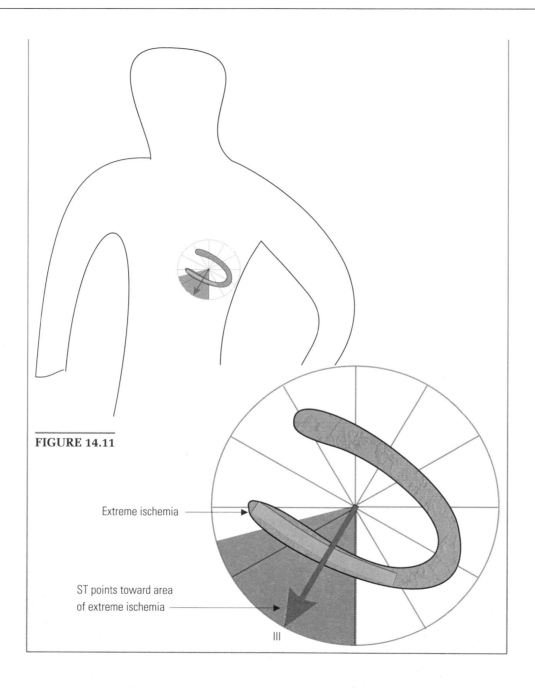

FIGURE 14.11

Extreme ischemia

ST points toward area
of extreme ischemia

III

Inferior STEMI: Reciprocal Changes

Transmural ischemia of the inferior wall attracts the ST segment toward the inferior wall. This produces ST segment elevation in the inferior leads, leads III and AVF, and usually lead II as well (Figure 14.11). The observers or leads on the other side of the heart also see the transmural process, but they see it as going away from them. Therefore, leads I and AVL show ST segment depression (Figure 14.12). This ST segment depression does not represent additional subendocardial ischemia of the lateral wall. There is no way for the ST segment to point towards the inferior wall without also pointing away from the lateral lead observers. This geometric fact of life is called reciprocal changes. It occurs in lateral transmural ischemia, and anterior transmural ischemia as well.

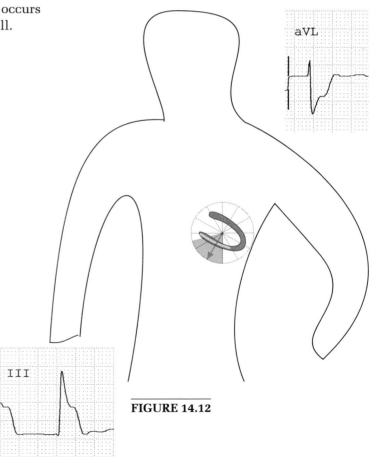

FIGURE 14.12

Inferior STEMI: Involvement of the Posterior Wall

Transmural ischemia of the inferior wall attracts the ST segment toward the inferior wall. This produces ST segment elevation in the inferior leads, leads III and AVF, and usually lead II as well. The ST depression in leads I and AVL are the result of reciprocal changes from the inferior process. The anterior leads in inferior transmural ischemia sometimes demonstrate ST segment depression. Below, a side view of the heart from a hypothetical lateral view (from the patient's left side) shows inferior transmural ischemia. The sensor in lead V2 sees this process as going away from it, and this can explain the ST segment depression in lead V2. The transmural ischemia in this example is not just inferior, but posterior as well. (There is also a chance that the ST segment in V2 is pointing away from subendocardial ischemia of the anterior wall, but this adds another disease. "No one test answers all the questions.")

FIGURE 14.13

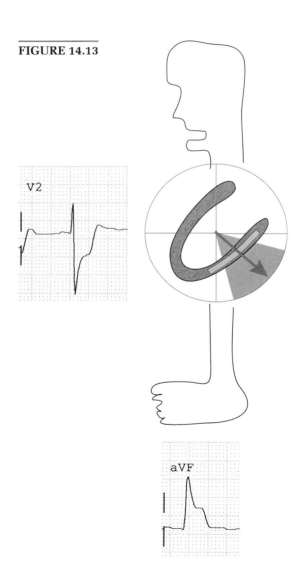

CASE EXAMPLE

2

STEMI: Syndrome of LAD Occlusion

EKG: The ST segment is elevated in two consecutive leads from V1, V2, V3, or V4 (Figure 14.14).

Visualization: The ST is pointing anteriorly toward the patient's septum, anterior wall, or inferior wall.

Critical Thinking: Since the ST segment is pointing toward the septal and anterior walls, we locate the area of extreme or transmural ischemia here. The left anterior descending coronary artery (LAD) supplies blood (Figure 14.19) to the septum through its septal perforators and the anterolateral wall through its diagonal branches. We expect a significant obstruction with a ruptured plaque and a superimposed thombus in the LAD. We apply the Third Rule of the T Waves. We ignore the T wave changes and ST depression and diagnose ST elevation myocardial infarction (NSTEMI). The LAD supplies nearly half the myocardium (Figure 14.18) with blood and so pump failure may result. This can lead to shock, pulmonary edema, or congestive heart failure. The LAD supplies the anterior part of the septum, so bundle branch block, hemiblock, or complete heart block may occur.

Pattern to Memorize

The ST waves point toward (+120° to +157.5°) in at least 2 of leads V1, V2, V3, and V4, producing ST elevation in these leads.

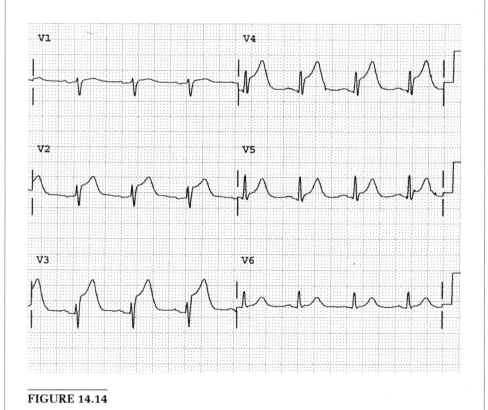

FIGURE 14.14

LBBB as an ST Elevation Equivalent

In the setting of symptoms suggestive of an acute coronary syndrome, a new left bundle branch block is equivalent to diagnosis of ST segment elevation myocardial infarction (STEMI). If the LBBB is not known to be old, it should be considered clinically identical to a new STEMI.

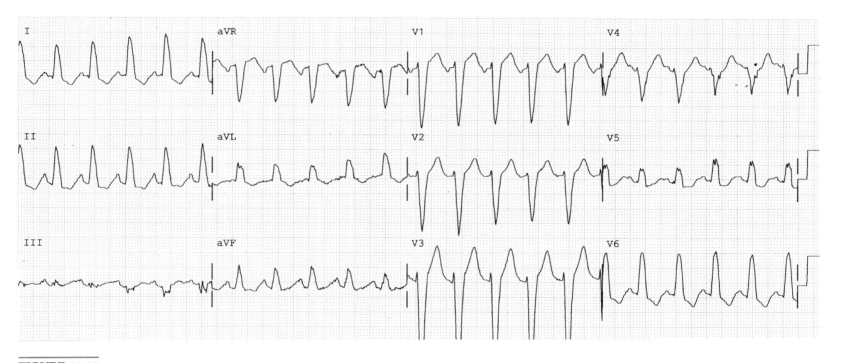

FIGURE 14.15

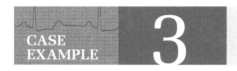

STEMI: Syndrome of Circumflex Artery Occlusion

EKG: The ST segment is positive in leads I and AVL (Figure 14.16).

Visualization: The ST is pointing to the patient's left side toward the lateral wall (Figure 14.17).

Critical Thinking: Since the ST segment is pointing toward the lateral wall (Figure 14.16), we locate the area of extreme or transmural ischemia here (Figure 14.17). The left circumflex coronary artery (LCX) supplies blood to the lateral wall through its obtuse marginal branches. In 10% of patients it supplies a branch to the AV node, and then the inferior wall as well. We expect a significant obstruction with a ruptured plaque and a superimposed thombus in the LCX. We apply the Third Rule of the T Waves. We ignore the T wave changes and ST depression and diagnose ST elevation myocardial infarction (NSTEMI). The LCX supplies the AV node only 10% of the time, therefore heart block such as 1° AV block, Wenckebach, or complete heart block are much less common than with an RCA occlusion. The circumflex artery supplies a relatively smaller portion of the LV than does the LAD, so pump failure, shock, and systolic heart failure are less common.

MEMORIZE THIS!   **Pattern to Memorize**

The ST waves point toward (0° to −75°) in leads I and AVL, producing ST elevation in these leads.

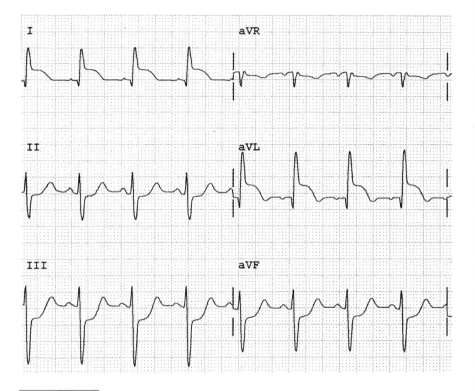

FIGURE 14.16

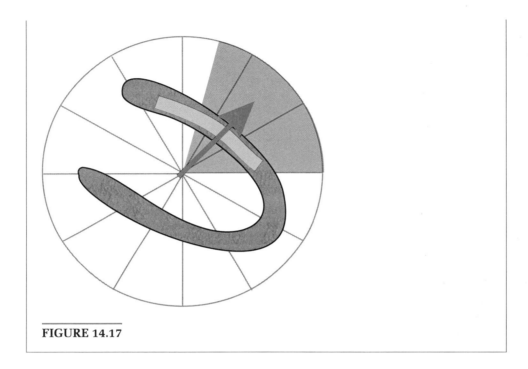

FIGURE 14.17

Complications of STEMI

Because of the total deprivation of oxygen supply many myocardial cells quickly become severely hypoxic and "stunned." Although possibly not yet irreversibly damaged, they can lose contractile function to the point of shock, pulmonary edema, or congestive heart failure, as the cells become functionally incapable without oxygen for energy. Many cells die, and they die quickly. Mechanical complications such as rupture of the ventricular septum, rupture of the free wall of the left ventricle, rupture of the mitral valve papillary muscle, and aneurysm formation can occur. Infarction of the septum can damage the right and left bundle branches leading to heart block.

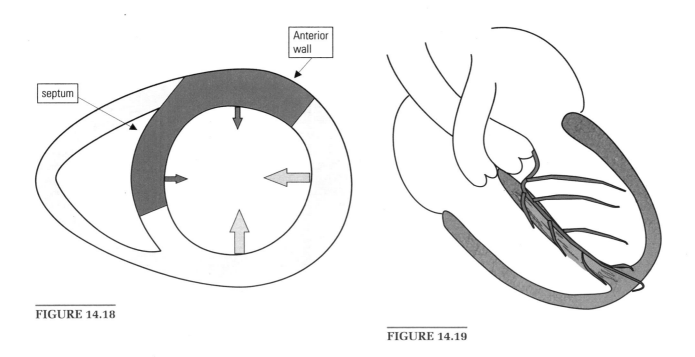

FIGURE 14.18

FIGURE 14.19

TABLE 14.1 Location of the ST Segments: Patterns to Memorize

Patterns of ST Segment Elevation	Location of Ischemia/Infarction
III, AVF (+/− II)	Inferior
I, AVL	Lateral
I, II, AVF	Apical
V1, V2	Septal
V3, V4	Anterior
V5, V6	Lateral

SAMPLE COMPLETED WORKSHEET

BASIC MEASUREMENTS			EVALUATION FOR ISCHEMIA OR INFARCTION	
Parameter	Measurement	Interpretation	Abnormal Parameter	If present, note the leads (or location) that contain the abnormality
HR	56	Abnormal	Inverted T waves	
Rhythm	Sinus bradycardia	Abnormal	ST depression	
PR	0.16	Normal		
QRS	0.08	Normal	ST elevation	Inferior
QT	0.34		Q waves or equivalent	
QTc	0.33	Short		
P direction	Normal	Normal		
QRS direction	Normal	Normal		

Instructions for Chapter 14 Worksheets

A) Complete basic measurements.
B) Note if ST Elevation is present in two or more leads that represent a pattern in Table 14.1. Describe this as ST elevation MI (STEMI) and note the location. In addition, Rule three of the T waves applies. ST elevation takes precedence over any associated T wave inversion or ST segment depression.
C) Provide an interpretation.

Clinically Based Critical Thinking: Interpretation

Since ST elevation is present in II, III, and AVF, read STEMI and localize it to the inferior wall. Rule three of the T waves applies. Ignore the ST depression in I and AVL, which represent reciprocal changes. The ST elevation is the significant finding. The artery to the inferior wall (usually RCA) is occluded. Therapy to open it is indicated as soon as possible. Short QT may be congenital or acquired and related to drug or electrolytes effect. Sinus bradycardia is common in the setting of acute inferior wall MI.

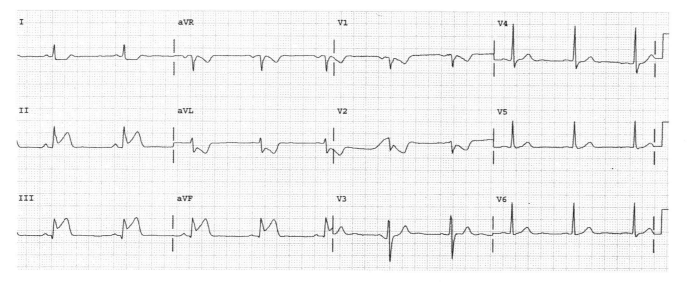

BASIC MEASUREMENTS			EVALUATION FOR ISCHEMIA OR INFARCTION	
Parameter	**Measurement**	**Interpretation**	**Abnormal Parameter**	**If present, note the leads (or location) that contain the abnormality**
HR			Inverted T waves	
Rhythm			ST depression	
PR				
QRS			ST elevation	
QT			Q waves or equivalent	
QTc				
P direction				
QRS direction				

Instructions for Chapter 14 Worksheets

A) Complete basic measurements.
B) Note if ST Elevation is present in two or more leads that represent a pattern in Table 14.1. Describe this as ST elevation MI (STEMI) and note the location. In addition, Rule three of the T waves applies. ST elevation takes precedence over any associated T wave inversion or ST segment depression.
C) Provide an interpretation.

Clinically Based Critical Thinking: Interpretation

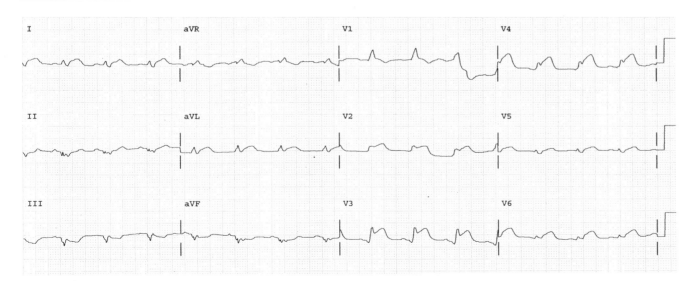

BASIC MEASUREMENTS			EVALUATION FOR ISCHEMIA OR INFARCTION	
Parameter	Measurement	Interpretation	Abnormal Parameter	If present, note the leads (or location) that contain the abnormality
HR			Inverted T waves	
Rhythm			ST depression	
PR				
QRS			ST elevation	
QT			Q waves or equivalent	
QTc				
P direction				
QRS direction				

Instructions for Chapter 14 Worksheets

A) Complete basic measurements.
B) Note if ST Elevation is present in two or more leads that represent a pattern in Table 14.1. Describe this as ST elevation MI (STEMI) and note the location. In addition, Rule three of the T waves applies. ST elevation takes precedence over any associated T wave inversion or ST segment depression.
C) Provide an interpretation.

Clinically Based Critical Thinking: Interpretation

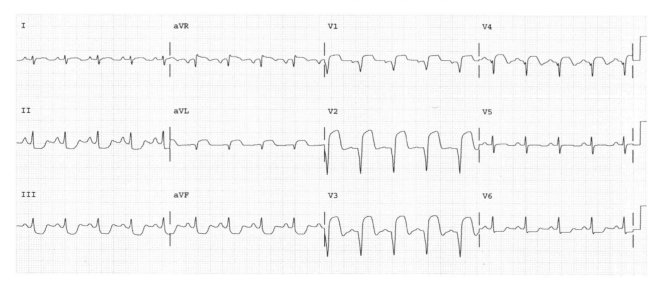

BASIC MEASUREMENTS			EVALUATION FOR ISCHEMIA OR INFARCTION	
Parameter	Measurement	Interpretation	Abnormal Parameter	If present, note the leads (or location) that contain the abnormality
HR			Inverted T waves	
Rhythm			ST depression	
PR				
QRS			ST elevation	
QT			Q waves or equivalent	
QTc				
P direction				
QRS direction				

Instructions for Chapter 14 Worksheets

A) Complete basic measurements.
B) Note if ST Elevation is present in two or more leads that represent a pattern in Table 14.1. Describe this as ST elevation MI (STEMI) and note the location. In addition, Rule three of the T waves applies. ST elevation takes precedence over any associated T wave inversion or ST segment depression.
C) Provide an interpretation.

Clinically Based Critical Thinking: Interpretation

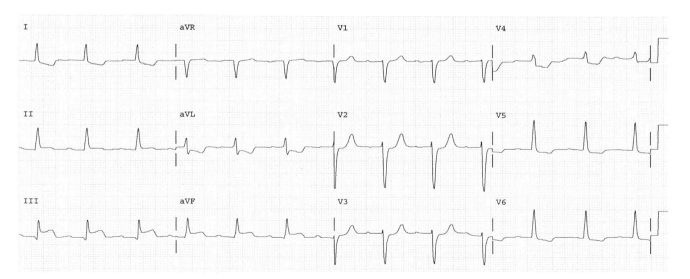

263

Prolonged Arterial Occlusion: Q Waves and Equivalents

The Three Parts of the QRS

The QRS complex represents depolarization of the ventricles. There are three separate times and three different ways that the QRS direction must be visualized. In Chapter 10, the overall direction of the entire QRS was used to diagnose hemiblock. In Chapters 11 and 12, visualization of the very end of the QRS provided the diagnosis of right versus left bundle branch block. Finally, the direction of the first 0.04 seconds is used to diagnose Q wave infarction. This must be evaluated on every EKG unless LBBB is present. The initial part of the QRS complex is one little box, or 0.04 seconds wide. Possibilities for this first part of the QRS are shown in Figure 15.1 a–c. Looking at only the first 0.04 seconds (or the first little box) of the QRS, Figure 15.1a is positive, Figure 15.1b is both positive and negative, and Figure 15.1c is negative.

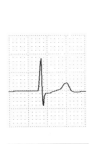 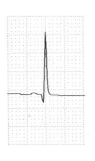 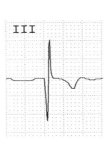

FIGURE 15.1a   **FIGURE 15.1b**   **FIGURE 15.1c**

The QRS: Beginning Normally

This initial part of the QRS normally distributes itself evenly and equally through all parts of the left ventricle. This can be visualized as pointing to the patient's left side and inferiorly.

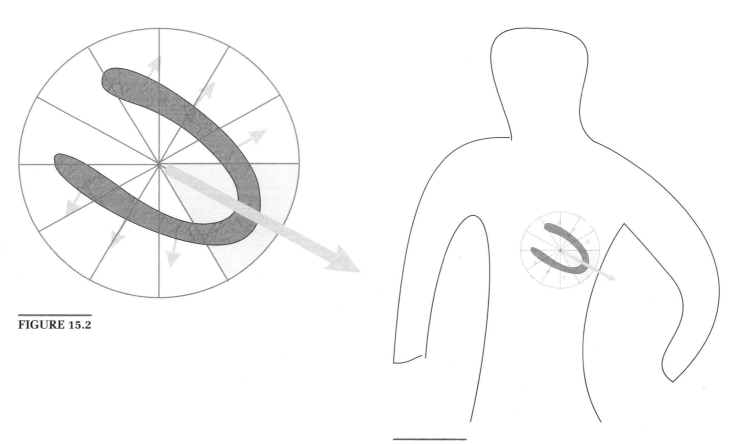

FIGURE 15.2

FIGURE 15.3

The QRS: Beginning Abnormally

Complete occlusion of an epicardial artery by a ruptured plaque and super-imposed thrombus causes extreme ischemia and ST segment elevation point-ing toward the involved area of the LV (see Chapter 14). When the obstruction is not relieved, death of a wide thickness of myocardial cells (transmural in-farction) results. The diagnostic hallmark of this transmural infarction on the EKG is an abnormality of the initial part of the QRS, which points away from the infarcted area. This dead tissue generates no electrical contribution to the QRS. The surviving parts of the ventricle produce a QRS that rotates away from the dead zone. This QRS beginning can be visualized as pointing away from an area of electrically dead myocardial cells. This negative beginning to the QRS is called a Q wave.

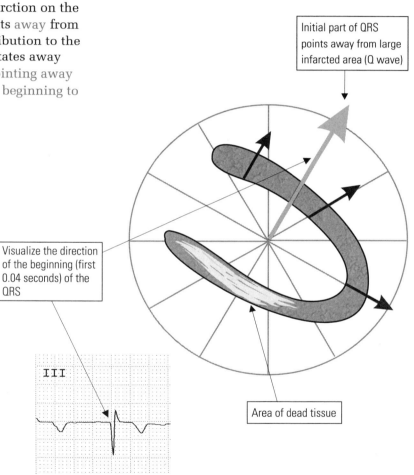

Initial part of QRS points away from large infarcted area (Q wave)

Visualize the direction of the beginning (first 0.04 seconds) of the QRS

III

Area of dead tissue

FIGURE 15.4

Criteria for Significant Q Waves

The criteria for an abnormal beginning to the QRS is that the first 0.04 seconds is on average negative. Figure 15.5 demonstrates four QRS complexes, each with a Q wave. The first QRS (Letter A) in Figure 15.5 demonstrates the obvious case of an abnormal Q wave. The whole QRS is negative in this example. There is no question then that the first 0.04 seconds is negative and, therefore, forms a significant Q wave. The second QRS (Letter B) demonstrates a QRS that is positive and negative. Since the first 0.04 seconds though is entirely negative, this is also a significant Q wave. The third example in Figure 15.5 (Letter C) is the case that presents a problem clinically for the EKG reader. The first 0.04 seconds of the QRS is partly negative and partly positive. A useful terminology for this borderline case is nonspecific Q wave. The last QRS (Letter D) demonstrates a clearly positive initial 0.04 seconds even though it started with a Q wave. This is a normal Q wave.

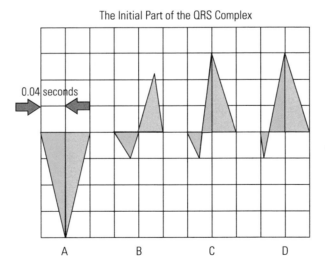

The Initial Part of the QRS Complex

0.04 seconds

A   B   C   D

FIGURE 15.5

Timing of Q Wave Infarction

Timing of the infarction can be suggested but not proven on a single EKG. If an abnormal Q wave pattern is present, the timing can be characterized according to Table 15.1. The presence of ST segment elevation always suggests acuteness (hours) of the event, particularly if it is the first EKG obtained (Figure 15.6a). After a few hours or days, ST segment elevation can end in an inverted T wave, as in Figure 15.6b. After a period of days to weeks, the ST elevation usually resolves into T wave inversion, as in Figure 15.6c. After a month or so, the T wave may completely normalize as in Figure 15.6d, and the infarction is termed either "old" or "age indeterminate." In addition, if this is the only EKG, the First Rule of the T Waves still applies. These T waves may be a separate event, represent ischemia or infarction, and may be new or old.

TABLE 15.1

T wave/ST pattern	Timing estimate
ST elevation	Acute
ST depression	Recent
T wave iInversion	Recent
Normal T and ST segments	Old, or age indeterminate

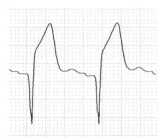

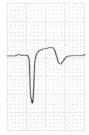

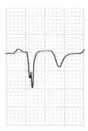

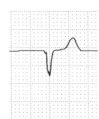

FIGURE 15.6a   **FIGURE 15.6b**   **FIGURE 15.6c**   **FIGURE 15.6d**

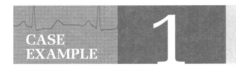

Inferior Q Wave Infarction

EKG: The first 0.04 seconds of the QRS are entirely negative in leads II, III, and AVF. These are significant Q waves.

Visualization: The beginning of the QRS is pointing to the left and superiorly away from the inferior wall.

Critical Thinking: The beginning of the QRS is pointing away from the inferior wall (Figure 15.7). We expect an infarction to be present in the inferior wall of the left ventricle. This is permanent loss of cells. The right coronary artery (RCA) supplies blood to the inferior and posterior walls. We expect a significant obstruction with either a plaque (or a plaque plus a clot) in that artery. Timing of the infarction can be suggested but not proven. Since there are inverted T waves, this suggests that the Q waves may be relatively acute or recent. Additionally, if this is the only EKG, the First Rule of the T Waves still applies. These T waves may be related to the Q wave infarction, and time it as recent. Or these T waves may represent new ischemia or infarction

Pattern to Memorize: Q waves point away (−45° to −90°) from leads II, III and AVF.

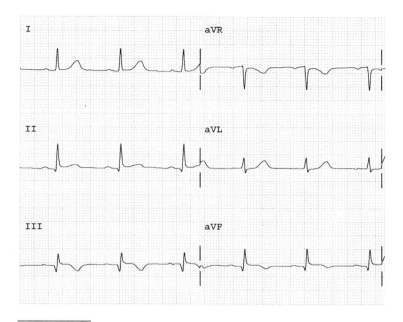

FIGURE 15.7

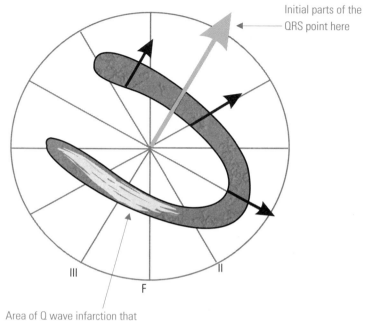

Initial parts of the QRS point here

Area of Q wave infarction that resulted from untreated STEMI

Septal and Anterior Wall Infarction

CASE
EXAMPLE

2

EKG: The first 0.04 seconds of the QRS are on average negative in leads V1, V2, and V3. These are Q wave equivalents (Figure 15.8).

Visualization: The beginning of the QRS is pointing to the left and posteriorly away from the septal and anterior walls.

Critical Thinking: The beginning of the QRS is pointing away from the septal and anterior walls. We expect an infarction to be present in the septal and anterior walls of the left ventricle. This is permanent loss of cells. The left anterior descending branch (LAD) of left coronary artery (LCA) supplies blood to the septal and anterior walls. We expect a significant obstruction with either a plaque (or a plaque plus a clot) in that artery. Timing of the infarction can be suggested but not proven. Since there are normal T waves, this suggests that the Q waves may be old, and the exact age indeterminate.

Pattern to Memorize: Q waves point away (−22.5° to −60°) from leads V1, V2, and V3.

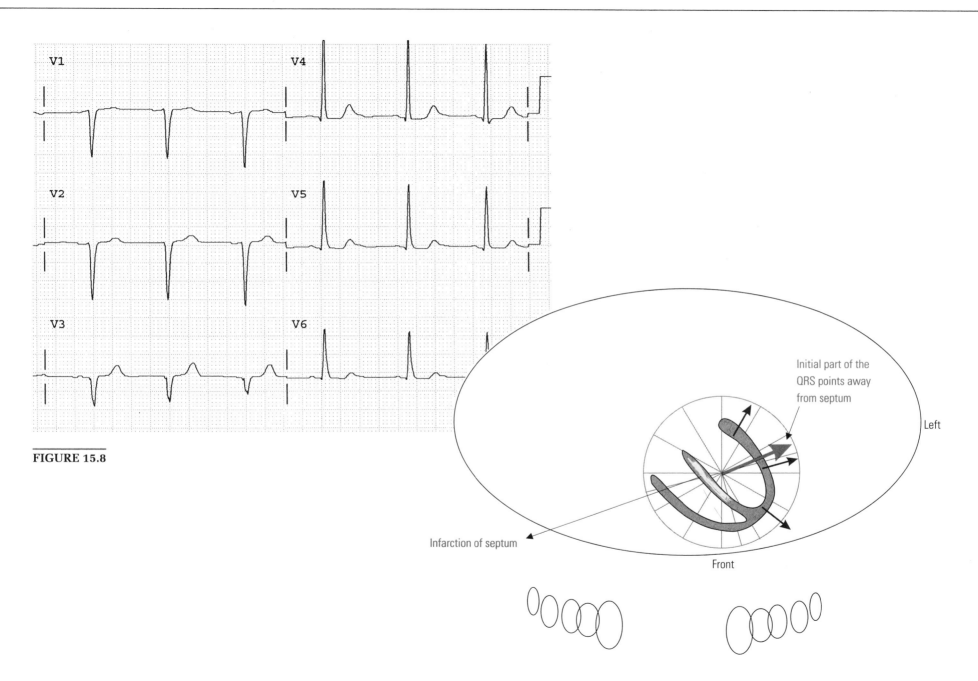

FIGURE 15.8

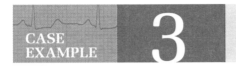

3 Septal Infarction with RBBB and LAHB

Septal infarctions are sometimes complicated by conduction disturbances. The right and left bundle branches are located within the myocardial layer of the ventricular septum. When the septum is damaged, the bundle branches or parts of them may be damaged as well. Importantly, RBBB does not affect the initial part of the QRS. Examine the example (Figure 15.9a).

a) The initial QRS shows significant Q waves in leads V1 through V4, indicating septal and anterior Q wave infarction.

b) The last part of the QRS points anterior and rightward, indicating RBBB.

c) The mean QRS in the frontal plane is upward (−90°), indicating LAHB.

d) A single lesion in the LAD caused the infarction that resulted in all the above.

The most common conduction problems associated with septal infarctions are RBBB, LBBB, RBBB and LAHB, RBBB and LPHB, 2° AV Block, and complete heart block. Except for isolated RBBB, the above conduction diseases may require a temporary ventricular pacemaker.

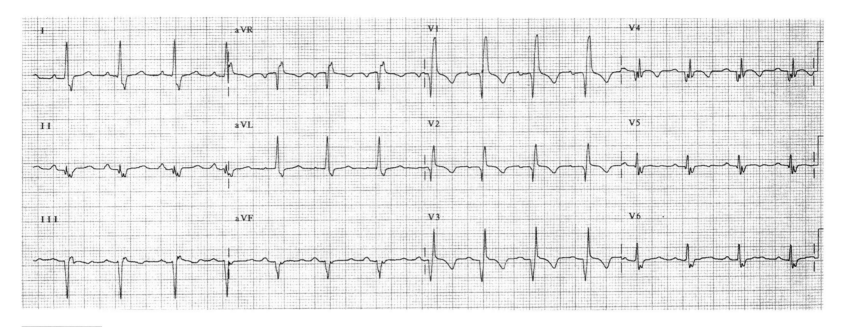

FIGURE 15.9a

4 Septal Infarction Causing LBBB

There is no reliable way to diagnose infarction or ischemia on the EKG in a patient with LBBB. **The patient in Figure 15.10 *may* have had a septal infarction as the cause of the LBBB. There is just no useful way to figure that out from the EKG. LBBB is LBBB. It indicates likely significant underlying pathology, but creates a "fog of war" that prevents the use of the EKG to help diagnose its cause.** The EKG below should *not* be read as septal infarction. It should *not* be read as transmural ischemia. It should be read as LBBB.

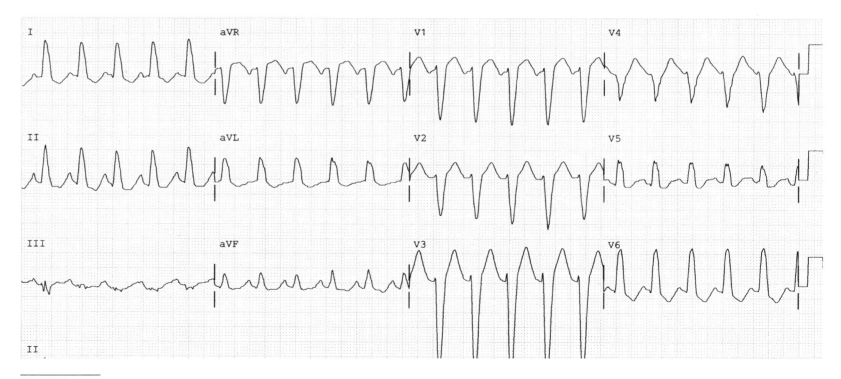

FIGURE 15.10

Less Specific Patterns of Infarction: Poor R Wave Progression

As in the inferior and lateral leads, leads V1, V2, and V3 can have an initial QRS that is intermediate between clearly abnormal and definitely normal. This borderline appearance is shown in Figure 15.11. There are several causes. Septal infarction can cause it, as can anything that decreases the ability of a sensor on the chest wall to record voltage. Some other clinical conditions that cause poor R wave progression are chronic lung disease, pericardial effusion, pneumothorax, and a large amount of breast tissue.

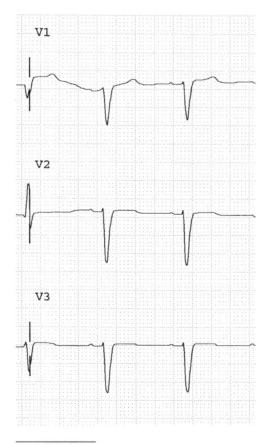

FIGURE 15.11

The Q Wave Equivalent: Inferior and Lateral Leads

Normal and abnormal Q waves were already discussed and illustrated in Figure 15.5. The QRS can still begin abnormally, even without the presence of a Q wave, as shown in Figure 15.12. Although the last QRS on the chart (Letter E) has no Q wave, the initial 0.04 seconds of the QRS is clearly negative. This is a Q wave equivalent and conveys the same information as a regular Q wave.

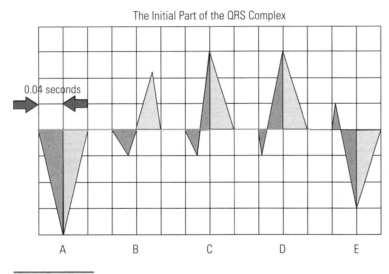

The Initial Part of the QRS Complex

0.04 seconds

A   B   C   D   E

FIGURE 15.12

The Q Wave Equivalent: Posterior Infarction

Figure 15.13 demonstrates a tall wide R wave in leads V1 and V2. The beginning of the QRS points away from the posterior wall. This is analgous to a Q wave for the posterior wall. Usually, as in this case, an inferior infarction is present on the EKG as well.

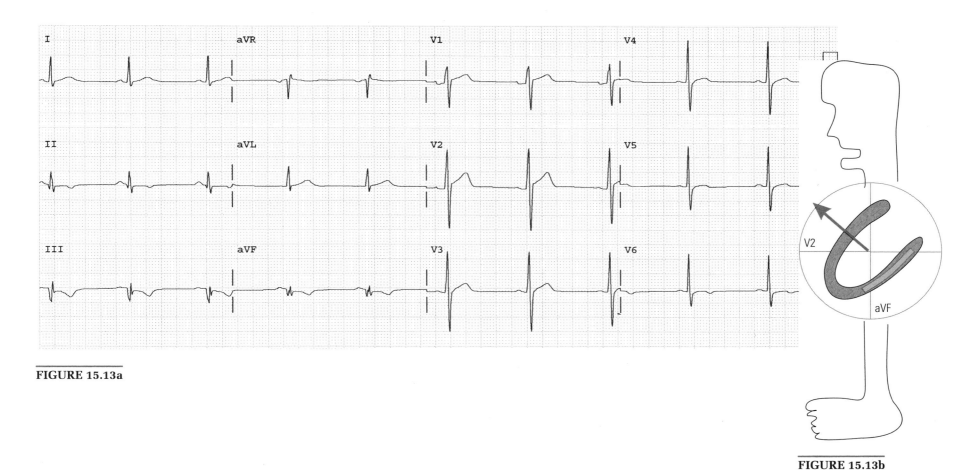

FIGURE 15.13a

FIGURE 15.13b

Summary of Criteria for Q Wave Infarction

TABLE 15.2

Q Wave Pattern	Location of Infarction
II, III, AVF	Inferior
I, AVL	Lateral
V1, V2	Septal
V3, V4	Anterior
V5, V6	Lateral
Tall wide R wave in V2	Posterior

SAMPLE COMPLETED WORKSHEET

BASIC MEASUREMENTS			EVALUATION FOR ISCHEMIA OR INFARCTION	
Parameter	Measurement	Interpretation	Abnormal Parameter	If present, note the leads (or location) that contain the abnormality
HR	72	Normal	Inverted T waves	Inferior and posterior
Rhythm	Sinus	Normal	ST depression	
PR	0.14	Normal		
QRS	0.09	Normal	ST elevation	
QT	0.40		Q waves or equivalent	Inferior and posterior
QTc	0.34	Normal		
P direction	Normal	Normal		
QRS direction	Normal	Normal		

Instructions for Chapter 15 Worksheets

A) Complete basic measurements.
B) Note if inverted T waves or ST segment depression is present. Note the presence of Q waves or Q wave equivalents as described in columns A, B, and E in Figure 15.12. Diagnose Q wave infarction according to the the patterns in Table 15.2. Next, attempt to estimate timing of the infarction according to the T and ST abnormalities by using Table 15.1 Lastly, interpret T or ST abnormality according to the 3 Rules of the T Waves.
C) Provide an interpretation.

Clinically Based Critical Thinking: Interpretation

Diagnose inferior infarction based on the Q Waves in the inferior leads. There is a wide R wave in leads V1 and V2, which is equivalent to a posterior wall Q wave. The inverted T waves in the inferior leads suggest that the infarction may have been recent. However if this is the only EKG, Rule 1 of the T Waves is in effect. The T inversion may be due to the previous Q wave infarction, but it may also be a new event! More information is necessary.

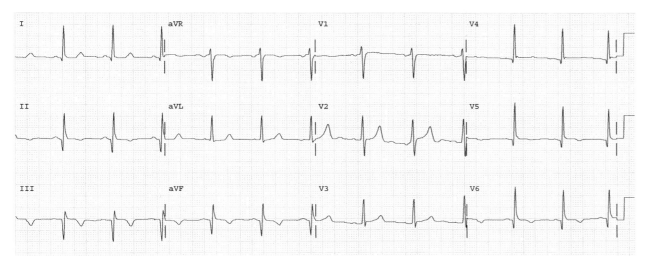

BASIC MEASUREMENTS			EVALUATION FOR ISCHEMIA OR INFARCTION	
Parameter	Measurement	Interpretation	Abnormal Parameter	If present, note the leads (or location) that contain the abnormality
HR			Inverted T waves	
Rhythm			ST depression	
PR				
QRS			ST elevation	
QT			Q waves or equivalent	
QTc				
P direction				
QRS direction				

Instructions for Chapter 15 Worksheets

A) Complete basic measurements.
B) Note if inverted T waves or ST segment depression is present. Note the presence of Q waves or Q wave equivalents as described in columns A, B, and E in Figure 15.12. Diagnose Q wave infarction according to the the patterns in Table 15.2. Next, attempt to estimate timing of the infarction according to the T and ST abnormalities by using Table 15.1 Lastly, interpret T or ST abnormality according to the 3 Rules of the T Waves.
C) Provide an interpretation.

Clinically Based Critical Thinking: Interpretation

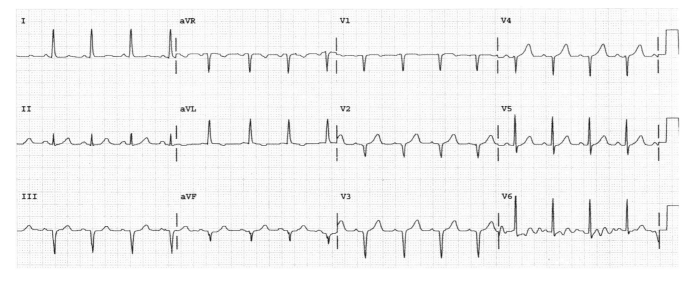

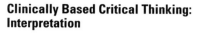

WORKSHEET 15.2

BASIC MEASUREMENTS			EVALUATION FOR ISCHEMIA OR INFARCTION	
Parameter	**Measurement**	**Interpretation**	**Abnormal Parameter**	**If present, note the leads (or location) that contain the abnormality**
HR			Inverted T waves	
Rhythm			ST depression	
PR				
QRS			ST elevation	
QT			Q waves or equivalent	
QTc				
P direction				
QRS direction				

Instructions for Chapter 15 Worksheets

A) Complete basic measurements.
B) Note if inverted T waves or ST segment depression is present. Note the presence of Q waves or Q wave equivalents as described in columns A, B, and E in Figure 15.12. Diagnose Q wave infarction according to the the patterns in Table 15.2. Next, attempt to estimate timing of the infarction according to the T and ST abnormalities by using Table 15.1 Lastly, interpret T or ST abnormality according to the 3 Rules of the T Waves.
C) Provide an interpretation.

Clinically Based Critical Thinking: Interpretation

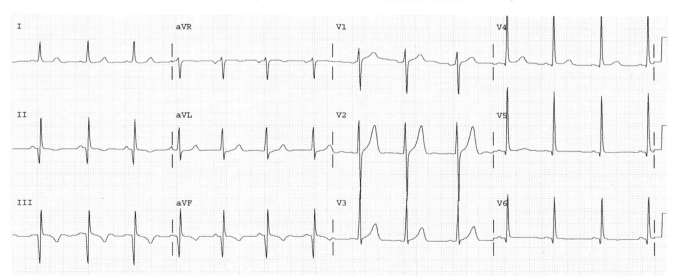

BASIC MEASUREMENTS			EVALUATION FOR ISCHEMIA OR INFARCTION	
Parameter	Measurement	Interpretation	Abnormal Parameter	If present, note the leads (or location) that contain the abnormality
HR			Inverted T waves	
Rhythm			ST depression	
PR				
QRS			ST elevation	
QT			Q waves or equivalent	
QTc				
P direction				
QRS direction				

Instructions for Chapter 15 Worksheets

A) Complete basic measurements.
B) Note if inverted T waves or ST segment depression is present. Note the presence of Q waves or Q wave equivalents as described in columns A, B, and E in Figure 15.12. Diagnose Q wave infarction according to the the patterns in Table 15.2. Next, attempt to estimate timing of the infarction according to the T and ST abnormalities by using Table 15.1 Lastly, interpret T or ST abnormality according to the 3 Rules of the T Waves.
C) Provide an interpretation.

Clinically Based Critical Thinking: Interpretation

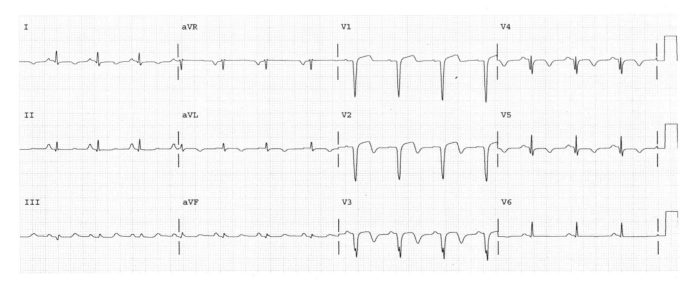

WORKSHEET V.1

BASIC MEASUREMENTS			EVALUATION FOR ISCHEMIA OR INFARCTION	
Parameter	**Measurement**	**Interpretation**	**Abnormal Parameter**	**If present, note the leads (or location) that contain the abnormality**
HR			Inverted T waves	
Rhythm			ST depression	
PR				
QRS			ST elevation	
QT			Q waves or equivalent	
QTc				
P direction				
QRS direction				

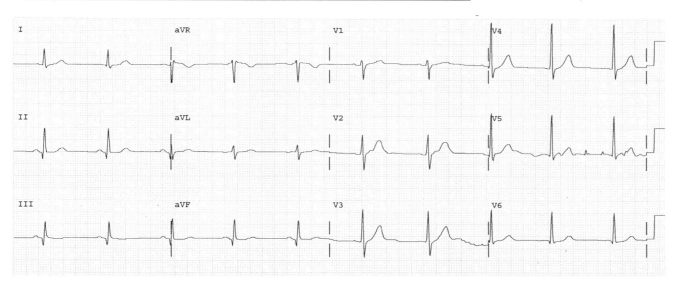

WORKSHEET V.2

BASIC MEASUREMENTS			EVALUATION FOR ISCHEMIA OR INFARCTION	
Parameter	Measurement	Interpretation	Abnormal Parameter	If present, note the leads (or location) that contain the abnormality
HR			Inverted T waves	
Rhythm			ST depression	
PR				
QRS			ST elevation	
QT			Q waves or equivalent	
QTc				
P direction				
QRS direction				

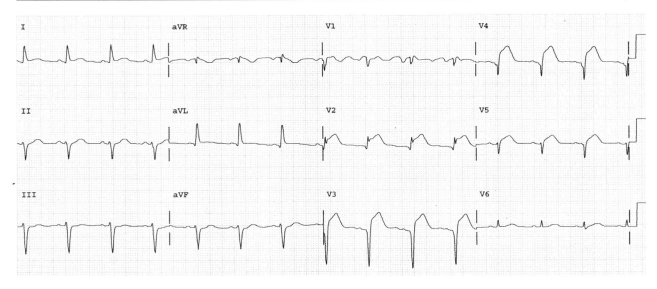

WORKSHEET V.3

BASIC MEASUREMENTS			EVALUATION FOR ISCHEMIA OR INFARCTION	
Parameter	Measurement	Interpretation	Abnormal Parameter	If present, note the leads (or location) that contain the abnormality
HR			Inverted T waves	
Rhythm			ST depression	
PR				
QRS			ST elevation	
QT			Q waves or equivalent	
QTc				
P direction				
QRS direction				

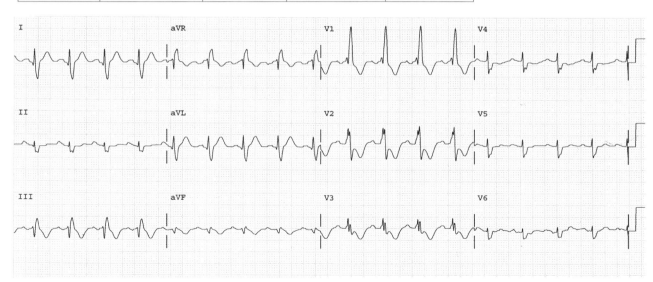

WORKSHEET V.4

BASIC MEASUREMENTS			EVALUATION FOR ISCHEMIA OR INFARCTION	
Parameter	Measurement	Interpretation	Abnormal Parameter	If present, note the leads (or location) that contain the abnormality
HR			Inverted T waves	
Rhythm			ST depression	
PR				
QRS			ST elevation	
QT			Q waves or equivalent	
QTc				
P direction				
QRS direction				

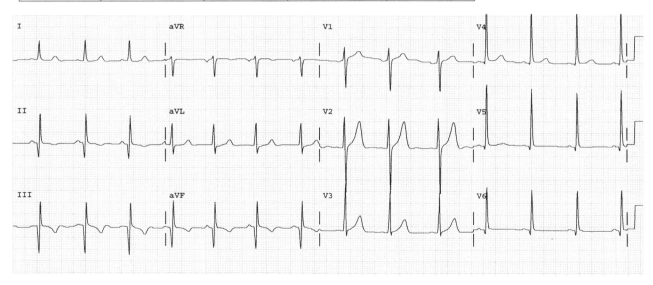

WORKSHEET V.5

BASIC MEASUREMENTS			EVALUATION FOR ISCHEMIA OR INFARCTION	
Parameter	Measurement	Interpretation	Abnormal Parameter	If present, note the leads (or location) that contain the abnormality
HR			Inverted T waves	
Rhythm			ST depression	
PR				
QRS			ST elevation	
QT			Q waves or equivalent	
QTc				
P direction				
QRS direction				

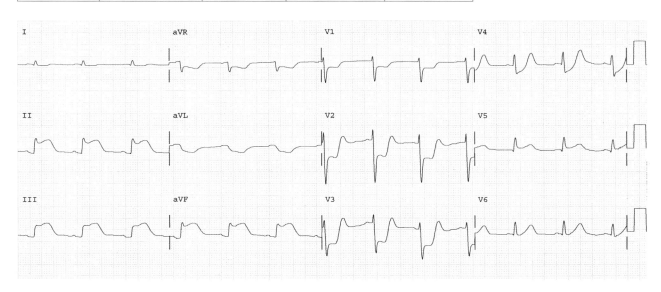

The Non-Ischemic Disorders: EKG Changes Related to Hypertrophy

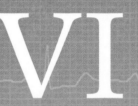

VI

Atrial Abnormalities

Self-Study Objectives

- Describe the normal right and left atrial anatomy
- Describe the pathophysiology of right atrial abnormality
- Identify right atrial abnormality on the EKG
- Describe the pathophysioogy of left atrial abnormality
- Identify left atrial abnormality on the EKG
- Describe the association of atrial abnormalities with valvular heart disease

Atrial Abnormalities: Anatomy

The right atrium (RA) is rightward and anterior. The left atrium (LA) is left-ward and posterior. The P wave represents atrial depolarization. Analysis and visualization of the P wave identify atrial abnormalities, or enlargement. Both right atrial abnormality (RAA) and left atrial abnormality (LAA) can be distinguished.

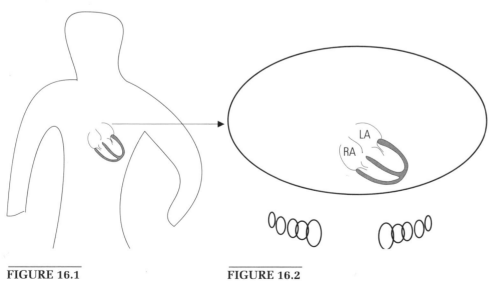

FIGURE 16.1   **FIGURE 16.2**

Right Atrial Abnormality: Pathophysiology

The right atrium is to the right and in front of the left atrium. In fact, the right atrium is the most rightward chamber of the heart. As the right atrium is subjected to the stress of either an increased pressure load or increased volume load, it enlarges as a compensatory mechanism to handle the increased work. Increased pressure in the right ventricle can be present from pulmonary hypertension secondary to chronic obstructive lung disease or pulmonary embolism. To handle the stiff muscular right ventricle, the right atrium has to "bulk up" in response. Increased volume in the right atrium can result from tricuspid regurgitation, commonly seen after pacemaker implantation, or because of long-standing pulmonary hypertension. To handle the volume overload, the right atrium has to "make space," and so it dilates.

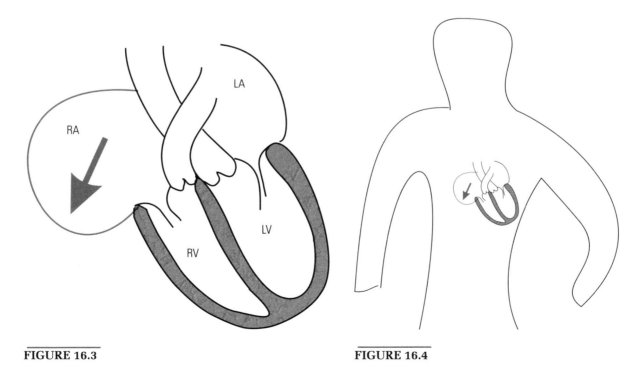

FIGURE 16.3   **FIGURE 16.4**

Right Atrial Abnormality: EKG Diagnosis

RAA can be diagnosed by an increase in the P wave amplitude to 2.5 little boxes in leads II, III, and AVF. RAA can also be diagnosed by a change in the P wave axis to a rightward direction. Right atrial abnormality on the EKG identifies enlargement in cavity size or muscle mass of the right atrium. Enlargement (bigger chamber) or hypertrophy (thicker walls) of the right atrium can change the P axis to a rightward direction. It can also increase the amplitude of the P wave.

A normal range for the P wave direction in the frontal plane is usually to the patient's left and inferior, although anywhere from −30 degrees to + 75 degrees may be normal. Visualization of the normal P wave should point in this range. A P wave direction of +90° to +105° or more indicates right atrial abnormality (RAA).

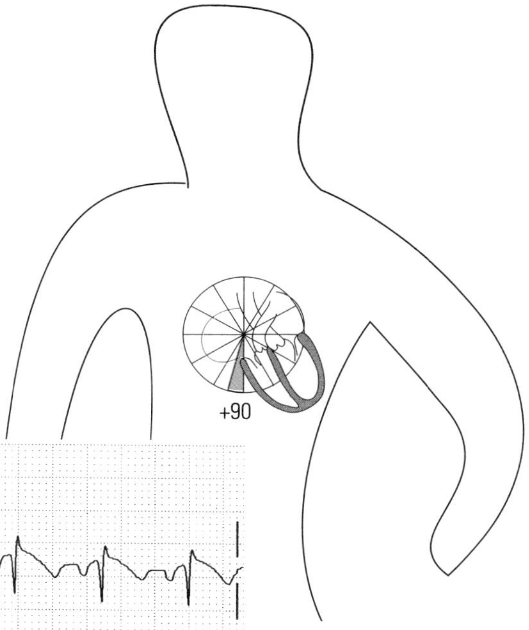

FIGURE 16.5

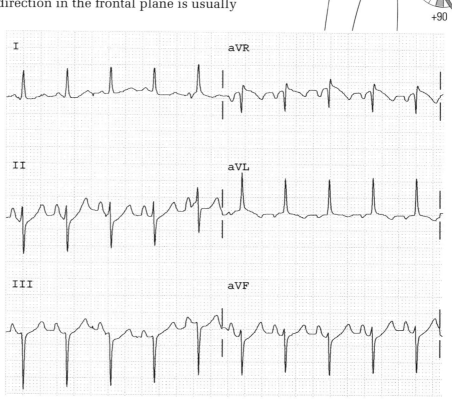

FIGURE 16.6

Left Atrial Abnormality: Pathophysiology

The left atrium is located behind the right atrium. In fact the left atrium is the most posterior chamber of the heart. As the left atrium is subjected to the stress of pressure or volume, it enlarges as a compensatory mechanism to handle the increased work. Increased pressure in the left ventricle can be present from hypertension, aortic stenosis, or hypertrophic obstructive cardiomyopathy. To handle the stiff muscular left ventricle, the left atrium has to "bulk up" in response. Increased pressure in the left atrium can directly result from mitral stenosis. Increased volume in the left atrium can result from mitral regurgitation. To handle the volume overload, the left atrium has to "make space," and so it dilates. The small pouch like sack attached to the left atrium is called the left atrial appendage. It is a critical structure clinically because it can harbor thrombus formation in low flow states, such as atrial fibrillation. Part of the thrombus can fragment and embolize to the systemic circulation, where it can cause stroke, bowel infarction, or limb embolus. Left atrial abnormality is a tiny part of the EKG that provides important clinical clues about disease on the left side of the heart.

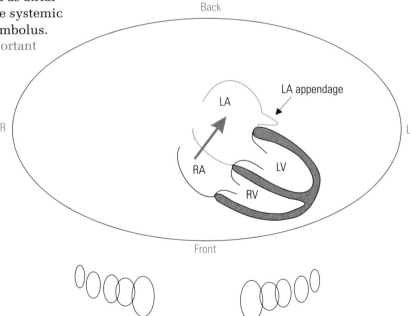

FIGURE 16.7

Left Atrial Abnormality: EKG Diagnosis

The direction of normal left atrial depolarization is posterior. The atrial depolarization force is represented on the EKG by the P wave. An increase in left atrial mass will increase the left atrium component of the P wave. **Lead V1 is usually the best lead for determining whether the left atrium is enlarged.** A left atrial abnormality creates a visible negative part to the P wave in V1. **Since the left atrium is further away from the sinus node than the right atrium, the second half of the P wave usually represents the left atrial component.** In LAA, the P wave in V1 is negative by at least 1 little box. The negative part of the P wave in V1 must also be 1 little box wide (0.04 seconds) (Figure 16.9).

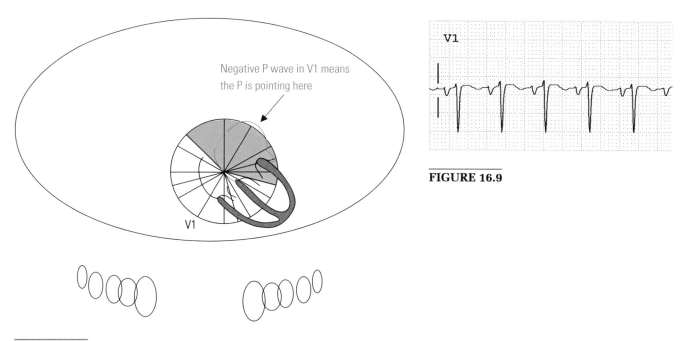

Negative P wave in V1 means the P is pointing here

V1

V1

FIGURE 16.9

FIGURE 16.8

Valvular Heart Disease

Diseased or malfunctioning heart valves cause increased burdens on the atria and ventricles (either volume or pressure) that can produce suggestive EKG changes. When valves leak (regurgitate) or become narrowed (stenose), they put a strain on at least one of the four chambers of the heart. This strain leads to increased mass of the involved chamber, as it tries to adapt to the added workload. The increased mass of any cardiac chamber creates a larger electrical force on the EKG, and this is how we detect hypertrophy of any of the heart chambers.

Regurgitation typically causes an added burden in the form of extra volume, which requires more space. The involved chambers of the heart respond by dilatation. This adaptation works well to offset the volume overload of regurgitation, as long as it develops slowly.

Stenosis is quite a different matter. It creates an added burden in the form of increased resistance to flow, which requires pressure generating ability. The involved chambers behind the stenosis typically develop thicker walls.

In the adult, the four most common valvular heart diseases that cause abnormalities on the EKG are mitral stenosis, mitral regurgitation, aortic regurgitation, and aortic stenosis.

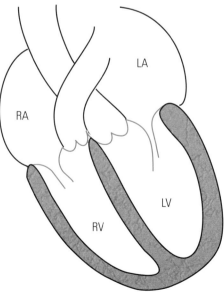

FIGURE 16.10

Mitral Stenosis

The mitral valve separates the left atrium from the left ventricle. When the valve is stenosed, it becomes constricted and narrows. This interferes with the flow of blood from the left atrium into the left ventricle. This increases the workload of the heart and eventually causes the left atrium to become enlarged. As the pressure backs up to the lungs, the right ventricle and right atrium also enlarge. Mitral stenosis is almost always a result of acute rheumatic fever. LAA, RVH, and RAA can be seen in mitral stenosis. The left ventricle is not involved. Treatment is surgical and is aimed at reducing the resistance to flow through the mitral valve.

Mitral stenosis causes blood to back up into the left atrium. It backs up from the left atrium into the lungs, causing shortness of breath (dyspnea). Eventually the blood backs up into the right ventricle and right atrium. The results are dilated left atrium, right ventricular hypertrophy, and right atrial hypertrophy.

Meanwhile, the left ventricle does not see any problem. There is no extra work for the left ventricle. Mitral stenosis does not affect the left ventricle!

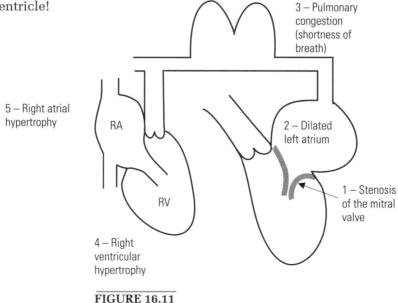

3 – Pulmonary congestion (shortness of breath)

5 – Right atrial hypertrophy

RA

2 – Dilated left atrium

1 – Stenosis of the mitral valve

RV

4 – Right ventricular hypertrophy

FIGURE 16.11

Mitral Regurgitation

Mitral regurgitation is most commonly caused by mitral valve prolapse, or rheumatic heart disease. Mitral regurgitation occurs when the mitral valve allows the backflow of blood from the left ventricle into the left atrium. The left atrium and left ventricle become dilated and hypertrophied trying to accommodate the extra blood volume. The EKG can demonstrate LAA and LVH.

Mitral regurgitation allows for a backward movement of blood between the left ventricle and left atrium during ventricular systole. The left atrium dilates to accommodate the extra blood volume. The left atrium fills from blood pumped from the right ventricle, but has no extra room to accommodate the regurgitant volume from the left ventricle. As a result, it dilates to compensate. The left ventricle dilates to accommodate the extra blood volume. The left ventricle fills with blood pumped from the right ventricle, but has no extra room to accommodate the regurgitant volume, and so it also dilates to compensate.

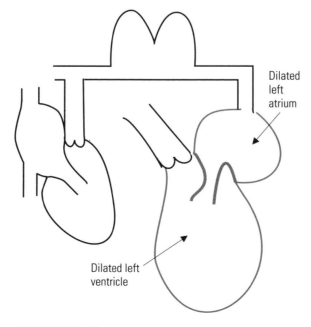

Dilated left atrium

Dilated left ventricle

FIGURE 16.12

SAMPLE COMPLETED WORKSHEET

BASIC MEASUREMENTS		
Parameter	**Measurement**	**Interpretation**
HR	125	Abnormal
Rhythm	Sinus tachycardia	Abnormal
PR	0.14	Normal
QRS	0.08	Normal
QT	0.32	
QTc	0.46	Long
P direction		Normal
QRS direction	superior	Not enough for LAHB

EVALUATION FOR ISCHEMIA OR INFARCTION	
T wave inversion	None
ST depression	None
ST elevation	None
Q waves or equivalent	Poor R wave progression

EVALUATION FOR SYSTEMIC EFFECTS: NOTE IF PRESENT	
LAA/RAA/LVH/RVH	LAA
Drug effect	
Hyper/ Hypokalemia	
Hyper/ Hypocalcemia	
Low voltage	
SI/QT III Pattern	
Pericarditis	

Instructions for Chapter 16 Worksheets

A) Make basic measurements and evaluate for ischemia and infarction.
B) Diagnose right or left atrial abnormality based on the criteria in Chapter 16.
C) Evaluate clinically.

Clinically Based Critical Thinking: Interpretation

Sinus tachycardia is present and suggests sympathetic stimulation. Medications and electrolyte values should be checked to explain the long QTc. Poor R wave progression could be the result of underlying infarction or lung disease. It is not a specific finding and needs to evaluated clinically. Left atrial abnormality is present which may be due to left ventricular disease such as hypertensive heart disease, or systolic or diastolic heart failure. LAA can also be associated with mitral stenosis or regurgitation.

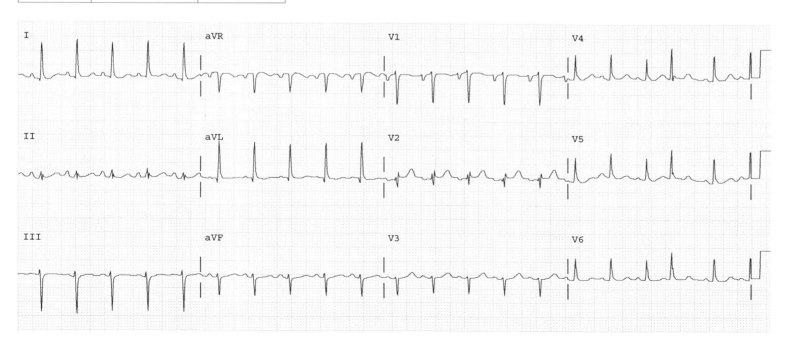

BASIC MEASUREMENTS			EVALUATION FOR ISCHEMIA OR INFARCTION		EVALUATION FOR SYSTEMIC EFFECTS: NOTE IF PRESENT	
Parameter	Measurement	Interpretation	T wave inversion		LAA/RAA/LVH/RVH	
HR			ST depression		Drug effect	
Rhythm			ST elevation		Hyper/ Hypokalemia	
PR			Q waves or equivalent		Hyper/ Hypocalcemia	
QRS						
QT					Low voltage	
QTc					SI/QT III pattern	
P direction					Pericarditis	
QRS direction						

Instructions for Chapter 16 Worksheets

A) Make basic measurements and evaluate for ischemia and infarction.
B) Diagnose right or left atrial abnormality based on the criteria in Chapter 16.
C) Evaluate clinically.

Clinically Based Critical Thinking: Interpretation

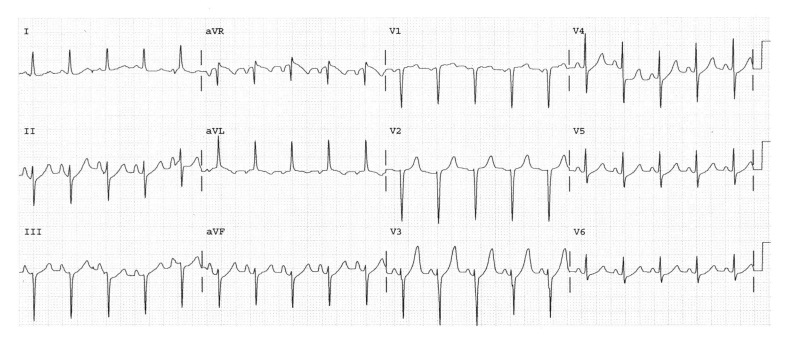

BASIC MEASUREMENTS			EVALUATION FOR ISCHEMIA OR INFARCTION		EVALUATION FOR SYSTEMIC EFFECTS: NOTE IF PRESENT	
Parameter	Measurement	Interpretation	T wave inversion		LAA/RAA/LVH/RVH	
HR			ST depression		Drug effect	
Rhythm			ST elevation		Hyper/ Hypokalemia	
PR			Q waves or equivalent		Hyper/ Hypocalcemia	
QRS					Low voltage	
QT					SI/QT III pattern	
QTc					Pericarditis	
P direction						
QRS direction						

A) Make basic measurements and evaluate for ischemia and infarction.
B) Diagnose right or left atrial abnormality based on the criteria in Chapter 16.
C) Evaluate clinically.

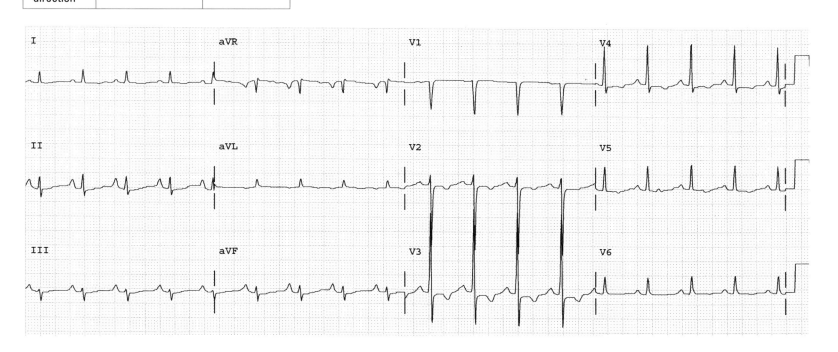

WORKSHEET 16.3

BASIC MEASUREMENTS			EVALUATION FOR ISCHEMIA OR INFARCTION		EVALUATION FOR SYSTEMIC EFFECTS: NOTE IF PRESENT	
Parameter	Measurement	Interpretation	T wave inversion		LAA/RAA/LVH/RVH	
HR			ST depression		Drug effect	
Rhythm			ST elevation		Hyper/ Hypokalemia	
PR			Q waves or equivalent		Hyper/ Hypocalcemia	
QRS						
QT					Low voltage	
QTc					SI/QT III pattern	
P direction					Pericarditis	
QRS direction						

Instructions for Chapter 16 Worksheets

Clinically Based Critical Thinking: Interpretation

A) Make basic measurements and evaluate for ischemia and infarction.

B) Diagnose right or left atrial abnormality based on the criteria in Chapter 16.

C) Evaluate clinically.

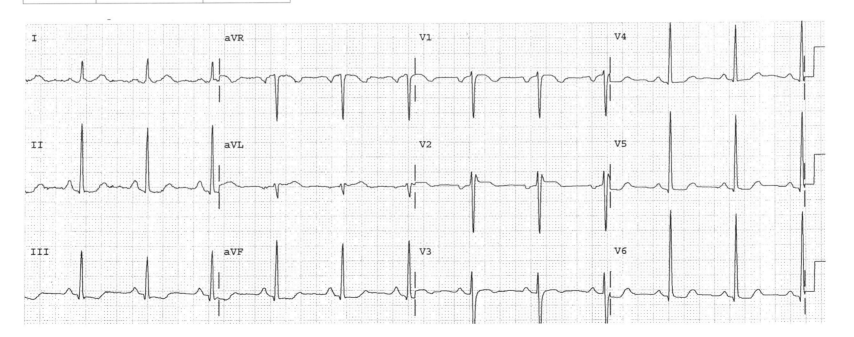

Left Ventricular Hypertrophy

17

Left Ventricular Hypertrophy: Overview

Left ventricular hypertrophy (LVH) refers to an increase in the wall thickness or dilation of the left ventricle. Left ventricular hypertrophy is often the result of increased pressure, or volume, within the left ventricular chamber. The left ventricle is located to the left and in back of the right ventricle. It is the systemic chamber of the heart and therefore is much larger in size than the right ventricle. Because the left ventricle is larger than the right ventricle, the overall QRS direction normally points posterior and leftward toward the left ventricle (Figure 17.2).

Self-Study Objectives

- Define and identify the following:

  The normal QRS direction

- Describe the pathophysiology of left ventricular hypertrophy

- Describe examples of pressure overload on the left ventricle

- Describe examples of volume overload on the left ventricle

- List criteria for the diagnosis of LVH on the EKG

- Identify LVH on the EKG

- Describe and identify ST changes in LVH

- Identify LVH simulating anterior wall infarction on the EKG

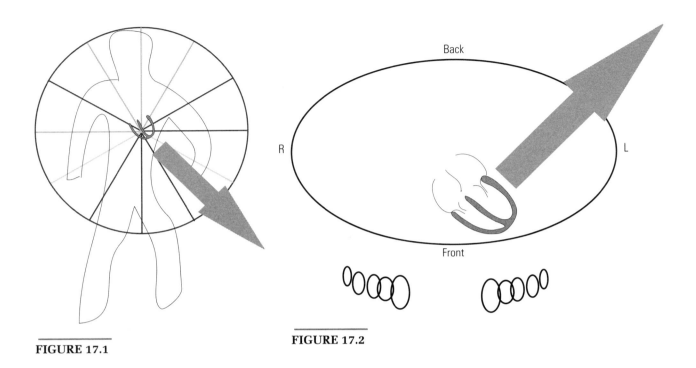

FIGURE 17.1   **FIGURE 17.2**

Left Ventricular Hypertrophy: Pathophysiology

Left ventricular hypertrophy (LVH) is often the result of an increase in pressure or volume within the left ventricle. When the pressure in the left ventricle increases, it adapts by developing a concentrically thicker wall (Figure 17.3). However, as the ventricular wall thickness increases, the actual cavity size becomes smaller. Increased pressure in the left ventricle is seen in systemic hypertension (HTN), aortic stenosis (AS), and hypertrophic obstructive cardiomyopathy (HOCM or IHSS). When the left ventricle is strained from volume overload, it compensates by making extra space or dilating (Figure 17.4). Volume overload is often seen in mitral or aortic regurgitation. LVH on the EKG indicates increased LV mass only. It does not distinguish between pressure overload and volume overload.

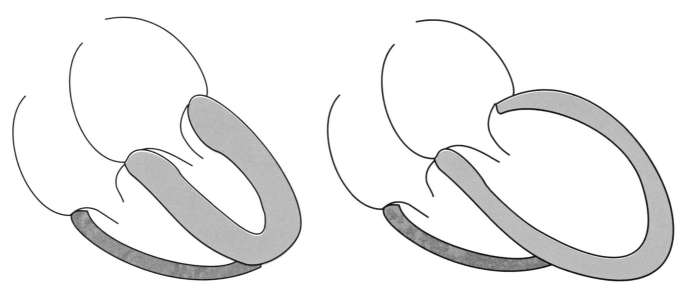

FIGURE 17.3   **FIGURE 17.4**

Volume Overload: Mitral and Aortic Regurgitation

Mitral regurgitation (MR) (see Chapter 16) occurs when the mitral valve allows the backflow of blood from the left ventricle into the left atrium. The left atrium and left ventricle become dilated and hypertrophied trying to accommodate the extra blood volume (Figure 17.5). Aortic regurgitation (AR) (Figure 17.6) causes a similar problem. The aortic valve lies between the left ventricle and the aorta. If the aortic valve does not close properly, blood leaks back into the left ventricle from the aorta. Because the left ventricle is receiving blood from both the left atrium and aorta, it stretches and eventually becomes enlarged. This results in left ventricular hypertrophy. The most common causes of aortic regurgitation are hypertension and rheumatic heart disease.

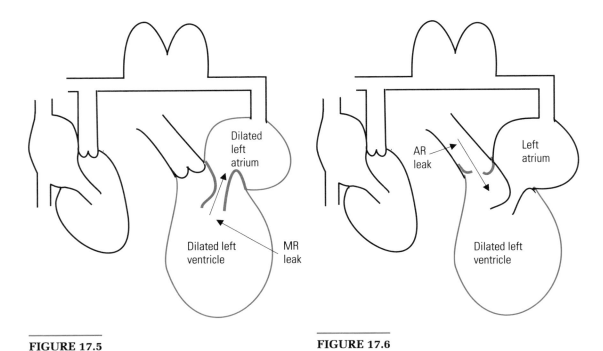

FIGURE 17.5   **FIGURE 17.6**

Pressure Overload: Hypertension and Outflow Obstruction

The most common cause of pressure overload is hypertension. **The presence of LVH on the EKG in the setting of hypertension establishes the presence of hypertensive heart disease and should prompt an investigation for other manifestations of end organ damage because of hypertension.**

Aortic stenosis (AS) (Figure 17.7) is a less common cause of pressure overload, but should be suspected with LVH on the EKG in the absence of hypertension. **It develops when the opening of the aortic valve becomes narrowed, restricting the flow of blood out of the left ventricle. The left ventricle hypertrophies to provide the extra force to push the blood through the aortic valve. The most common causes of aortic stenosis are rheumatic heart disease, congenital malformation, or calcification of the bicuspid valve.**

In pressure overload of the left ventricle from any cause, the left atrium hypertrophies as well. **The left atrium "bulks up" to develop enough force to push blood into a thick, muscular, unrelaxed ventricle. Hypertrophic obstructive cardiomyopathy (HOCM or IHSS) is a less common cause of LVH.**

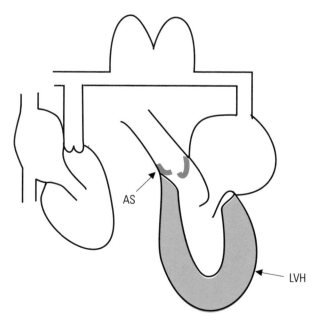

FIGURE 17.7

EKG Approach in LVH

Hypertrophy (Figure 17.8) of the left ventricle increases the amplitude of the left ventricular forces, because more mass generates more electricity. However the overall direction of the QRS is not really affected, as the left ventricular forces already predominate over the force generated simultaneously by the right ventricle. In the example of left ventricular hypertrophy in Figures 17.8

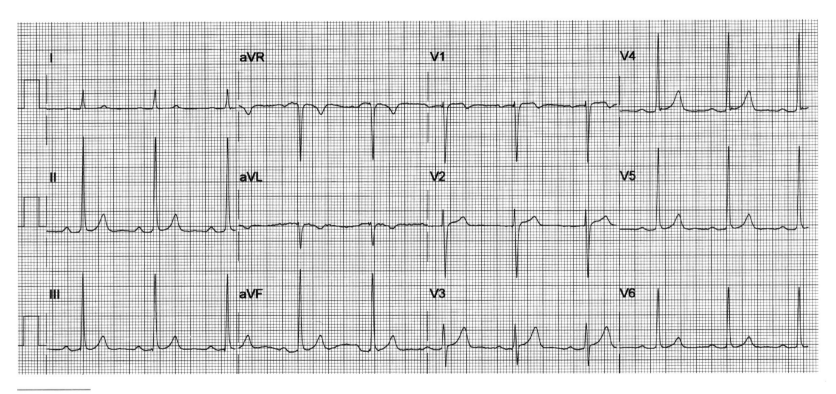

FIGURE 17.8

to 17.10, the mean QRS direction in the frontal and horizontal planes lies within the normal range, that is, to the patient's left and posterior. This is one of the cases where visualization of the direction of the force really does not help. The increased mass of the left ventricle (whether concentric with a small cavity or eccentric with a dilated cavity) increases the size (amplitude) of the QRS force. In LVH, the frontal plane, the horizontal plane, or both may show increased QRS amplitude. There are separate criteria for each plane.

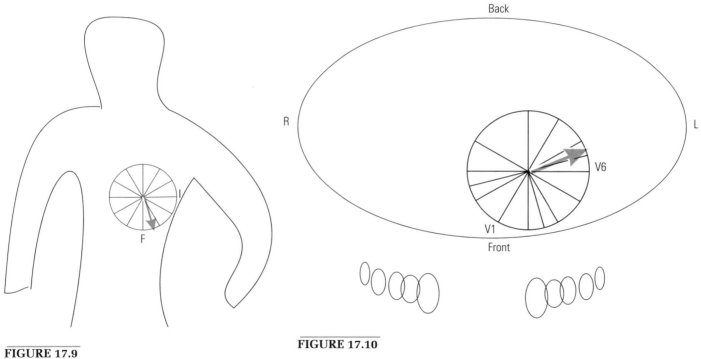

FIGURE 17.9

FIGURE 17.10

EKG Criteria for LVH in the Frontal Plane

Criteria: The depth of the S wave in lead III added to the height of the R wave in lead I equals 25 little boxes or more. (Here the sum is 31 little boxes.)

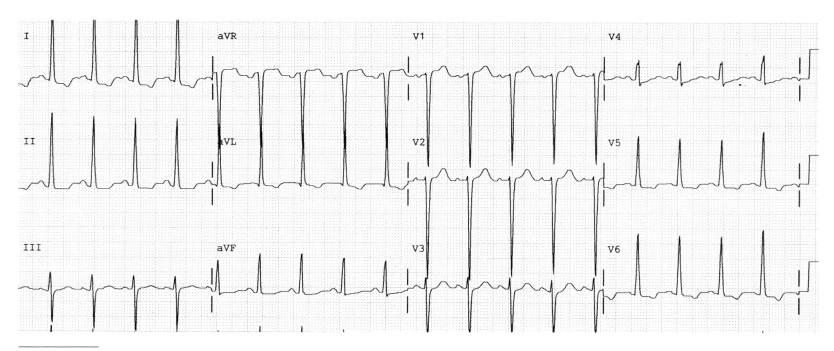

FIGURE 17.11

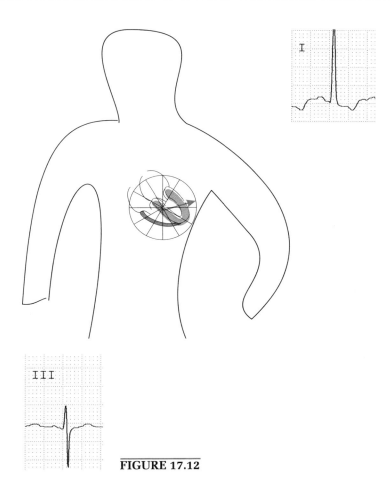

FIGURE 17.12

EKG Criteria for LVH in the Horizontal Plane

Criteria: The depth of the S wave in lead V1 added to the height of the R wave in lead V5 equals 35 little boxes or more. Here the sum is 44 little boxes.

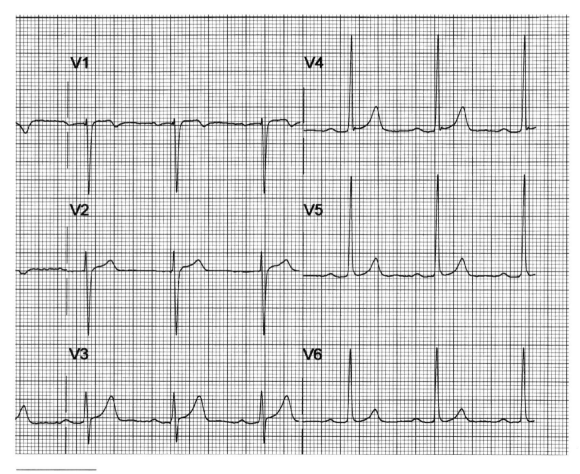

FIGURE 17.13

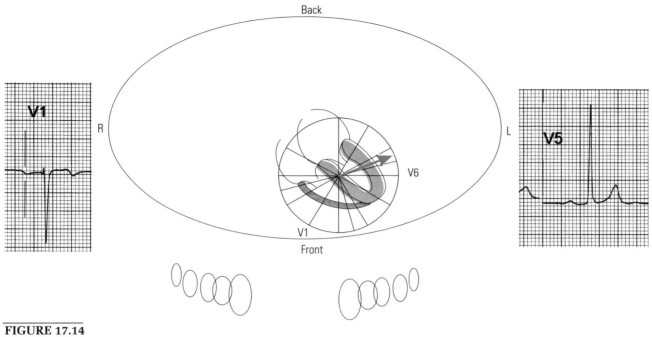

FIGURE 17.14

ST Segment Changes in LVH

In left ventricular hypertrophy (Figure 17.15), the ST segment may point opposite the mean QRS axis (Figure 17.16). This is sometimes referred to as
"strain pattern." These ST segment changes can be seen in the frontal plane,
the horizontal plane, or both. In either plane, the ST segment points away
from the left ventricle, as it would in left bundle branch block or subendocardial ischemia of the lateral wall. ST elevation in leads V1, and V2 may be
reciprocal changes due to the ST depression in the lateral leads, and not an
indication of transmural ischemia or infarction.

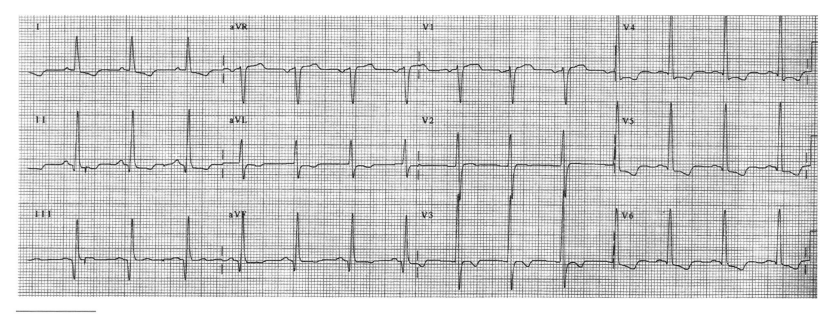

FIGURE 17.15

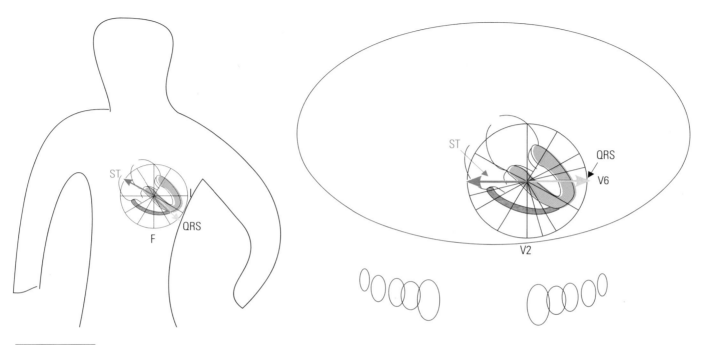

FIGURE 17.16

LVH Simulating Anterior Wall Infarction

As the left ventricle mass increases, it creates larger negative voltages in leads V1 and V2. A point can be reached at which the negative voltage washes out the R waves in these leads, giving the appearance of septal infarction. The Q wave equivalents in V1 and V2 may be due solely to LVH. The ST segment changes in LVH, which point away from the lateral walls, can cause the appearance of ST elevation, **simulating transmural ischemia of the inferior wall and septum.** On the other hand, hypertension frequently is the underlying cause of LVH, and hypertension is a major risk factor for coronary artery disease. LVH, by creating its own ST segment depression and elevation, as well as Q waves in the septal leads, complicates the interpretation of ischemia or infarction in these patients. Other tests and information are almost always necessary.

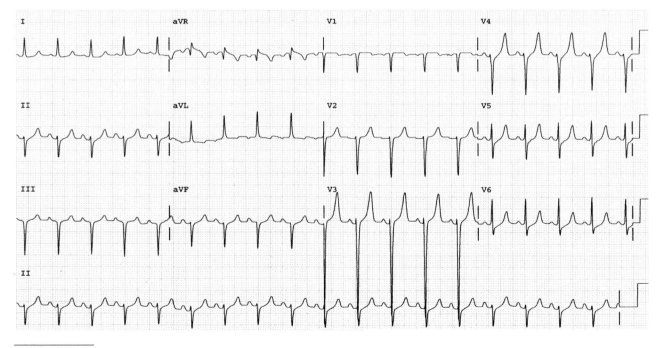

FIGURE 17.17

SAMPLE COMPLETED WORKSHEET

BASIC MEASUREMENTS		
Parameter	**Measurement**	**Interpretation**
HR	88	Normal
Rhythm	Sinus	Normal
PR	0.16	Normal
QRS	0.10	IVCD
QT	0.36	
QTc	0.44	
P direction		Normal
QRS direction	superior	Borderline LAHB

EVALUATION FOR ISCHEMIA OR INFARCTION	
T wave inversion	None
ST depression	Lateral
ST elevation	
Q waves or equivalent	V1 to V3

EVALUATION FOR SYSTEMIC EFFECTS: NOTE IF PRESENT	
LAA/RAA/LVH/RVH	LVH
Drug effect	
Hyper/ Hypokalemia	
Hyper/ Hypocalcemia	
Low voltage	
SI/QT III Pattern	
Pericarditis	

Instructions for Chapter 17 Worksheets

A) Make basic measurements, evaluate for ischemia and infarction, and atrial abnormality.
B) Diagnose LVH if criteria listed in Chapter 17 are present.
C) Evaluate clinically.

Clinically Based Critical Thinking: Interpretation

LVH is present by voltage since RI + SIII = 25. There are Q waves (this is not poor R wave progression; these are Q waves) in V1, V2 and V3, and so Q wave infarction criteria of the septum and anterior wall are present as well. A careful inspection of leads I, V5, and V6 shows ST segment depression, which may be due to LVH or to ischemia or infarction. Possible associations include hypertension, poorly controlled, with coexistent coronary disease.

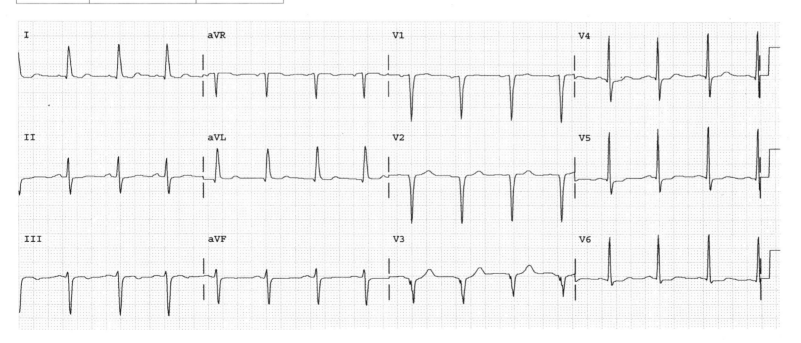

BASIC MEASUREMENTS			EVALUATION FOR ISCHEMIA OR INFARCTION		EVALUATION FOR SYSTEMIC EFFECTS: NOTE IF PRESENT	
Parameter	Measurement	Interpretation	T wave inversion		LAA/RAA/LVH/RVH	
HR			ST depression		Drug effect	
Rhythm			ST elevation		Hyper/ Hypokalemia	
PR			Q waves or equivalent		Hyper/ Hypocalcemia	
QRS						
QT					Low voltage	
QTc					SI/QT III pattern	
P direction					Pericarditis	
QRS direction						

Instructions for Chapter 17 Worksheets

A) Make basic measurements, evaluate for ischemia and infarction, and atrial abnormality.

B) Diagnose LVH if criteria listed in Chapter 17 are present.

C) Evaluate clinically.

Clinically Based Critical Thinking: Interpretation

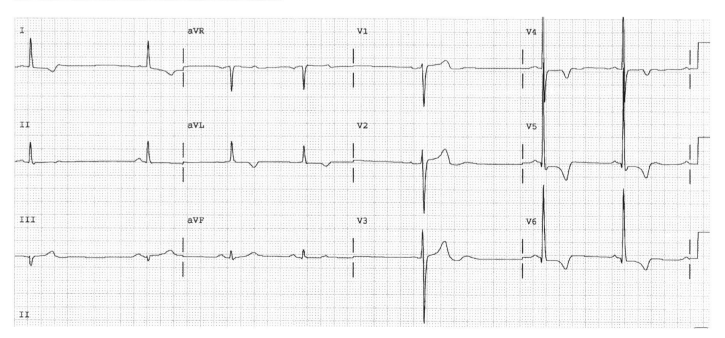

BASIC MEASUREMENTS			EVALUATION FOR ISCHEMIA OR INFARCTION		EVALUATION FOR SYSTEMIC EFFECTS: NOTE IF PRESENT	
Parameter	Measurement	Interpretation	T wave inversion		LAA/RAA/LVH/RVH	
HR			ST depression		Drug effect	
Rhythm			ST elevation		Hyper/ Hypokalemia	
PR			Q waves or equivalent		Hyper/ Hypocalcemia	
QRS						
QT					Low voltage	
QTc					SI/QT III pattern	
P direction					Pericarditis	
QRS direction						

Instructions for Chapter 17 Worksheets

A) Make basic measurements, evaluate for ischemia and infarction, and atrial abnormality.
B) Diagnose LVH if criteria listed in Chapter 17 are present.
C) Evaluate clinically.

Clinically Based Critical Thinking: Interpretation

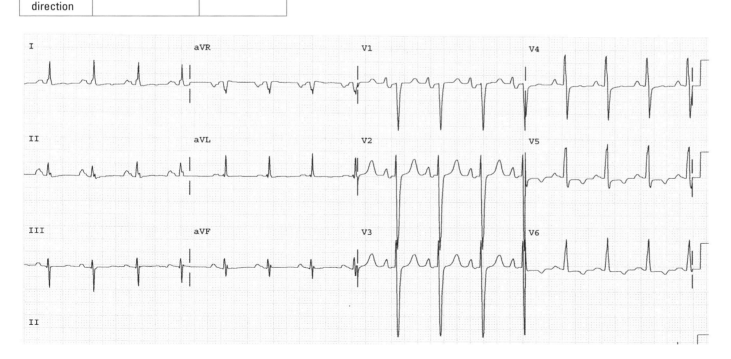

WORKSHEET 17.3

BASIC MEASUREMENTS			EVALUATION FOR ISCHEMIA OR INFARCTION		EVALUATION FOR SYSTEMIC EFFECTS: NOTE IF PRESENT	
Parameter	**Measurement**	**Interpretation**	T wave inversion		LAA/RAA/LVH/RVH	
HR			ST depression		Drug effect	
Rhythm			ST elevation		Hyper/ Hypokalemia	
PR			Q waves or equivalent		Hyper/ Hypocalcemia	
QRS						
QT					Low voltage	
QTc					SI/QT III pattern	
P direction					Pericarditis	
QRS direction						

A) Make basic measurements, evaluate for ischemia and infarction, and atrial abnormality.
B) Diagnose LVH if criteria listed in Chapter 17 are present.
C) Evaluate clinically.

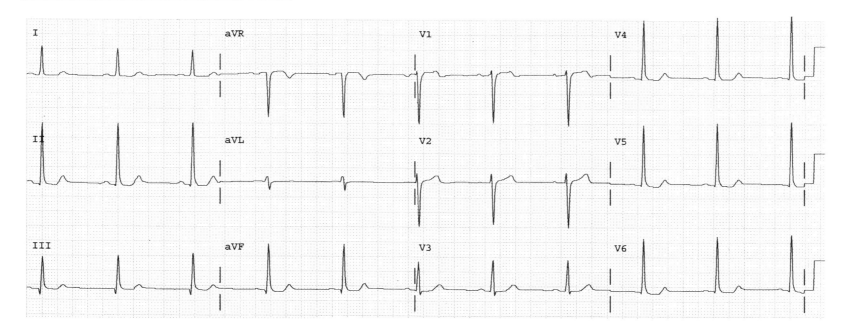

Right Ventricular Hypertrophy

Right Ventricular Hypertrophy: Overview

The normal QRS complex represents simultaneous depolarization of the right and left ventricles. Since the left ventricle is more massive than the right ventricle, the normal QRS direction is toward the left ventricle. Therefore, in the frontal plane, the normal QRS direction is to the patient's left (Figure 18.1). In the horizontal plane, the normal overall QRS direction also points to the left ventricle, which is to the patient's left and posterior (Figure 18.2). The diagnostic hallmark of right ventricular hypertrophy is an overall QRS direction that points either to the patient's right, anterior, or both (Figures 18.1 and 18.2).

Self-Study Objectives

- Define and identify the following:

  The normal QRS direction
- Describe the pathophysiology of right ventricular hypertrophy
- List the two criteria for diagnosing RVH on the EKG
- Identify RVH on the EKG
- Describe and identify ST changes in RVH
- Describe the EKG findings of RVH in chronic lung disease
- Describe the EKG findings of RVH in pulmonary embolism

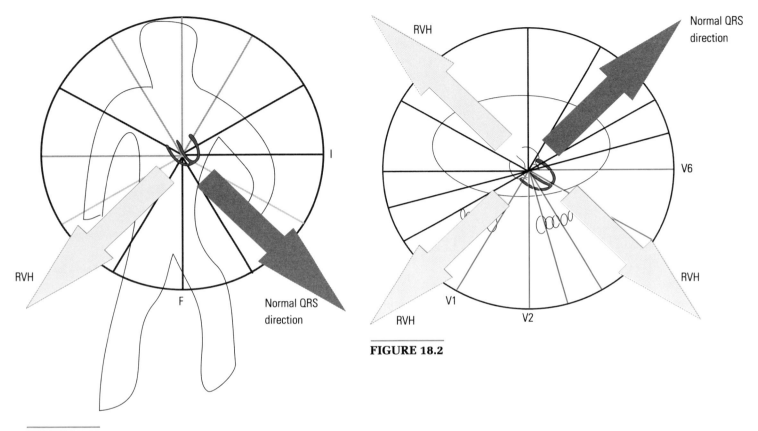

FIGURE 18.1

FIGURE 18.2

Right Ventricular Hypertrophy: Pathophysiology

As the right ventricle is subjected to the stress of pressure or volume, its mass increases as a compensatory mechanism to handle the increased work. Increased pressure in the right ventricle can be present from pulmonary hypertension. In adults, this is commonly due to obstructive lung disease or pulmonary emboli. The right ventricular adaptation is to increase its mass. Increased volume in the right ventricle can result from tricuspid regurgitation or an intracardiac shunt, such as an atrial septal defect (ASD). To handle the volume overload, the right ventricle has to "make space," and so it dilates.

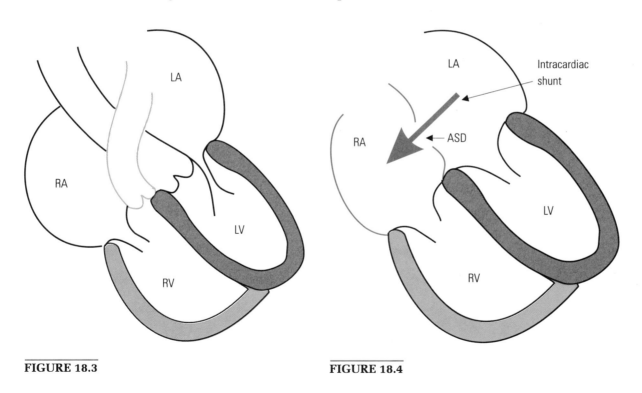

FIGURE 18.3

FIGURE 18.4

EKG Criteria for RVH in the Frontal Plane

The left ventricle is leftward and posterior. As it depolarizes simultaneously with the right ventricle, its more massive forces predominate. As a result, the mean QRS axis normally points toward the left ventricle. If the right ventricle can acheive enough mass to pull the mean QRS rightward in the frontal plane, then this indicates right ventricular hypertrophy. If lead I demonstrates the mean QRS axis in the frontal plane as rightward, this by itself indicates RVH. Chapter 8 demonstrated LPHB as an otherwise unexplained right axis. Now there is a differential diagnosis when an EKG has a mean QRS that points rightward: LPHB, RVH or a large lateral wall infarction. Other clues must be examined to help narrow down the diagnosis.

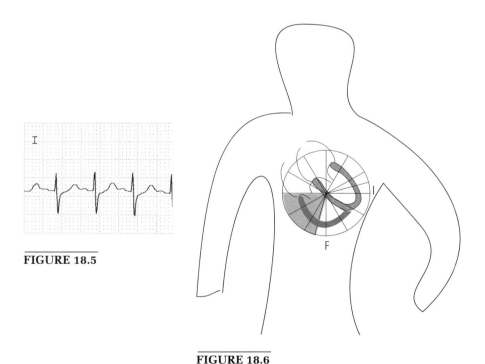

FIGURE 18.5

FIGURE 18.6

EKG Criteria for RVH in the Horizontal Plane

The left ventricle is leftward and posterior. As it depolarizes simultaneously with the right ventricle, its more massive forces predominate. As a result, the mean QRS axis normally points toward the left ventricle. If the right ventricle can acheive enough mass to pull the mean QRS either rightward or anterior, in either the frontal plane or the horizontal plane, then this indicates right ventricular hypertrophy. If lead I demonstrates the mean QRS axis in the frontal plane as rightward, this by itself indicates RVH. Notice that the mean QRS (in this example) in the horizontal plane is rightward and also anterior. Cut the right ventricle some slack. It is up against the left ventricle. If the right ventricle can pull the QRS either anterior or rightward, then this indicates RVH. (See Figure 6.63 for review)

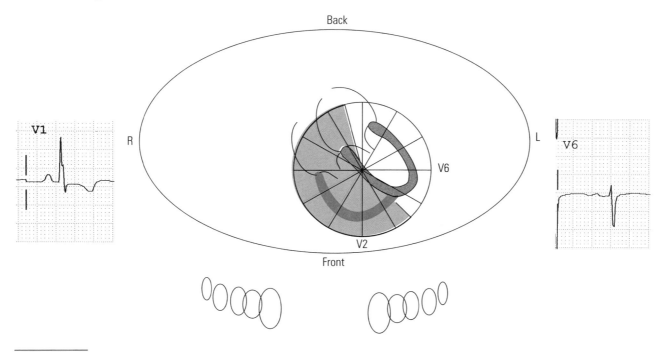

FIGURE 18.7

ST Segment Changes in RVH

In RVH (Figure 18.9), the ST segment or T wave axis may point away from the right ventricle. These ST or T wave changes can happen in the frontal plane, the horizontal plane, or both. In either plane, the ST or T points away from the right ventricle, as it would in right bundle branch block or subendocardial ischemia of the septum.

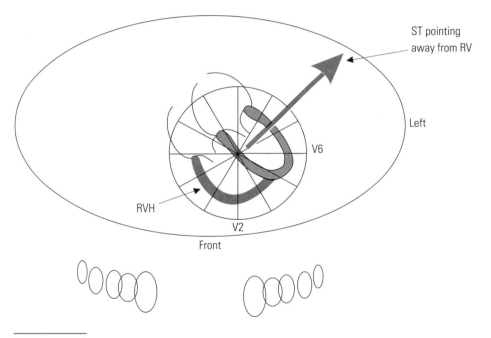

FIGURE 18.8

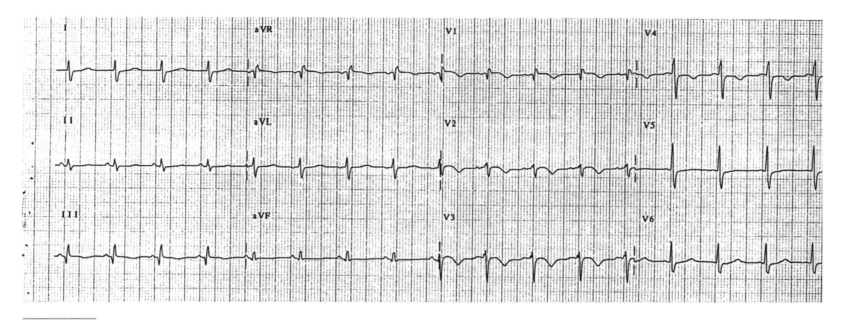

FIGURE 18.9

Obstructive Lung Disease

Obstructive lung disease (COPD), commonly caused by smoking, increases the pulmonary resistance to blood flow from the pulmonary artery. **When the resistance to blood flow rises, the pressure builds up in the right ventricle. The increased pressure must be generated by the right ventricle, which hypertrophies to meet the new increased workload.** The right atrium eventually becomes involved, as the right ventricle struggles to meet its new burdens. **The EKG shows RVH and RAA (Figure 18.11). COPD traps a large volume of air inside the lungs. This air is a terrible conductor of electricity and interferes with the recording of the EKG.** This can cause *low voltage* to appear on the EKG (Figure 18.11).

COPD reduces the cross-sectional area of blood flow through the lungs (Figure 18.10). This increases the pressure in the pulmonary artery, which the right ventricle must match and exceed, or the pulmonary valve would never open. The right atrium hypertrophies as well to assist the right ventricle meet its new workload.

When the level of trapped air gets severe, the EKG shows low voltage (Figure 18.11). If the sum of the QRS amplitude in leads I, II and III is less than 15 little boxes, low voltage is present. If none of the QRS complexes in leads V1, V2, or V3 is 15 little boxes by itself, then low voltage is present.

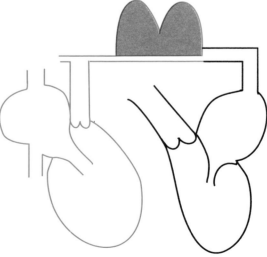

FIGURE 18.10

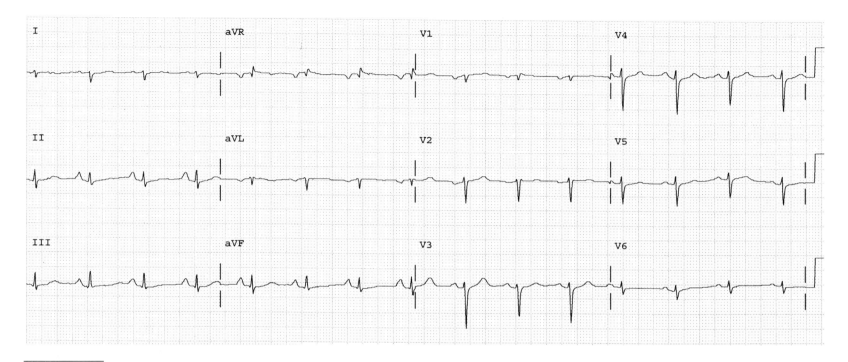

FIGURE 18.11

Pulmonary Embolism

Pulmonary embolism is usually part of a disease process termed venous thromboembolism (VTE). Because of a hypercoagulable state, trauma to a blood vessel, or low flow states, a thrombus can form in the venous system and then embolize to the pulmonary artery. Pulmonary embolism can develop as a single event, but it can also become recurrent. The embolus in the pulmonary artery obstructs blood flow to part of the lungs and increases the pressure behind the clot. The right ventricle typically dilates rapidly in response to this. In the acute setting, the EKG can (but may not) demonstrate sinus tachycardia, RVH, and RAA. If the pressure overload is severe, there can be a supply and demand mismatch for the right ventricle, and abnormal T waves can result. The EKG can show a T axis that points posterior, not away from the septum, but away from the free wall of the right ventricle, as illustrated in Figures 18.2 and 18.3 (also review Figure 6.63). The presence of an S wave in Lead I, with a Q wave and inverted T wave in Lead III is called SIQTIII, and is classic for pulmonary embolism.

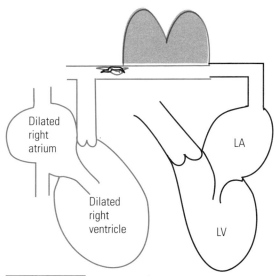

Dilated right atrium

Dilated right ventricle

LA

LV

FIGURE 18.12

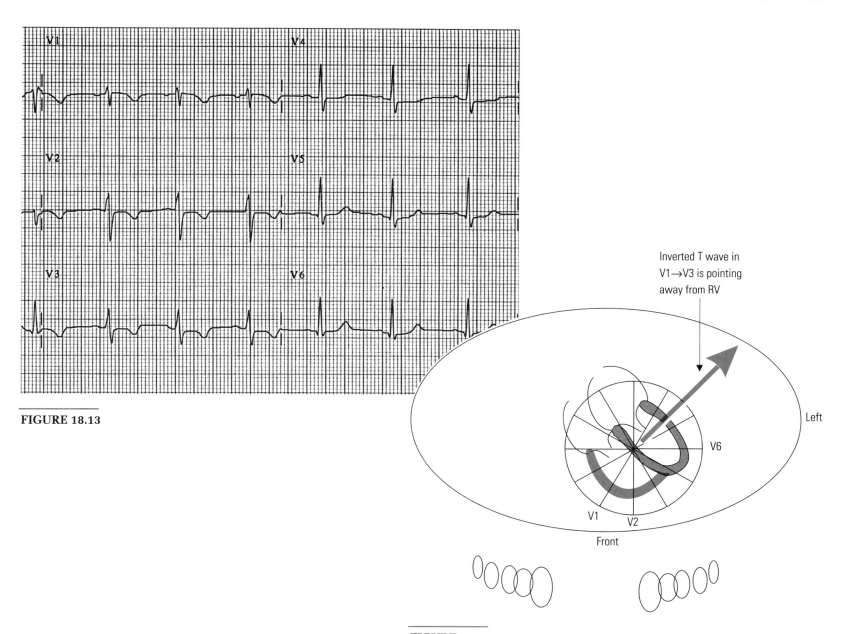

FIGURE 18.13

Inverted T wave in V1→V3 is pointing away from RV

Left

V6

V1   V2

Front

FIGURE 18.14

SAMPLE COMPLETED WORKSHEET

BASIC MEASUREMENTS			EVALUATION FOR ISCHEMIA OR INFARCTION		EVALUATION FOR SYSTEMIC EFFECTS: NOTE IF PRESENT	
Parameter	**Measurement**	**Interpretation**	T wave inversion		LAA/RAA/LVH/RVH	RVH
HR	115	Abnormal	ST depression		Drug effect	
Rhythm	Sinus tachycardia	Abnormal	ST elevation		Hyper/ Hypokalemia	
PR	0.14	Normal	Q waves or equivalent		Hyper/ Hypocalcemia	
QRS	0.08	Normal				
QT	0.28				Low voltage	
QTc	0.440				SI/QT III Pattern	
P direction		Normal			Pericarditis	
QRS direction	superior	Rightward RVH				

Instructions for Chapter 18 Worksheets

A) Make basic measurements, evaluate for ischemia and infarction, and atrial abnormality.
B) Diagnose RVH if the QRS direction is either rightward, anterior, or both.
C) Evaluate clinically.

Clinically Based Critical Thinking: Interpretation

Sinus tachycardia is present and represents increased sympathetic activity. The QRS direction is rightward in the frontal plane (R<S). This could represent RVH or LPHB. The HR of 115 confirms the patient is acutely ill regardless of the diagnosis.

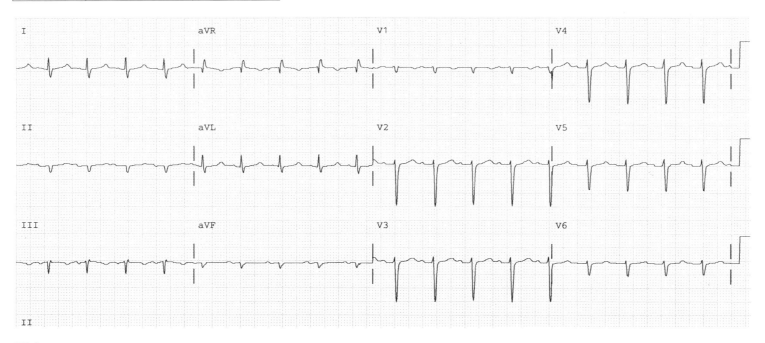

BASIC MEASUREMENTS			EVALUATION FOR ISCHEMIA OR INFARCTION		EVALUATION FOR SYSTEMIC EFFECTS: NOTE IF PRESENT	
Parameter	**Measurement**	**Interpretation**	T wave inversion		LAA/RAA/LVH/RVH	
HR			ST depression		Drug effect	
Rhythm			ST elevation		Hyper/ Hypokalemia	
PR			Q waves or equivalent		Hyper/ Hypocalcemia	
QRS						
QT					Low voltage	
QTc					SI/QT III pattern	
P direction					Pericarditis	
QRS direction						

Instructions for Chapter 18 Worksheets

A) Make basic measurements, evaluate for ischemia and infarction, and atrial abnormality.

B) Diagnose RVH if the QRS direction is either rightward, anterior, or both.

C) Evaluate clinically.

Clinically Based Critical Thinking: Interpretation

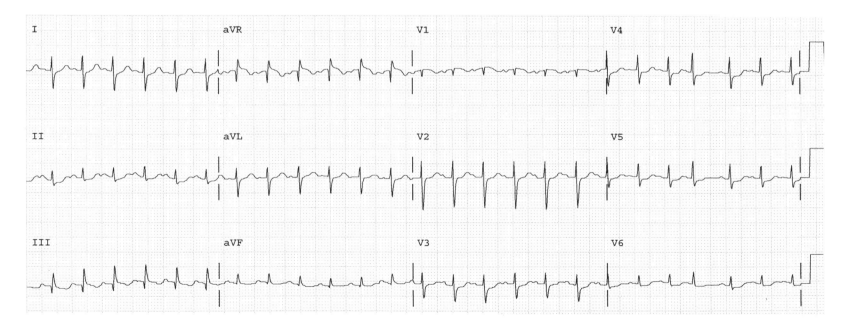

BASIC MEASUREMENTS			EVALUATION FOR ISCHEMIA OR INFARCTION		EVALUATION FOR SYSTEMIC EFFECTS: NOTE IF PRESENT	
Parameter	Measurement	Interpretation	T wave inversion		LAA/RAA/LVH/RVH	
HR			ST depression		Drug effect	
Rhythm			ST elevation		Hyper/ Hypokalemia	
PR			Q waves or equivalent		Hyper/ Hypocalcemia	
QRS						
QT					Low voltage	
QTc					SI/QT III pattern	
P direction					Pericarditis	
QRS direction						

Instructions for Chapter 18 Worksheets

A) Make basic measurements, evaluate for ischemia and infarction, and atrial abnormality.

B) Diagnose RVH if the QRS direction is either rightward, anterior, or both.

C) Evaluate clinically.

Clinically Based Critical Thinking: Interpretation

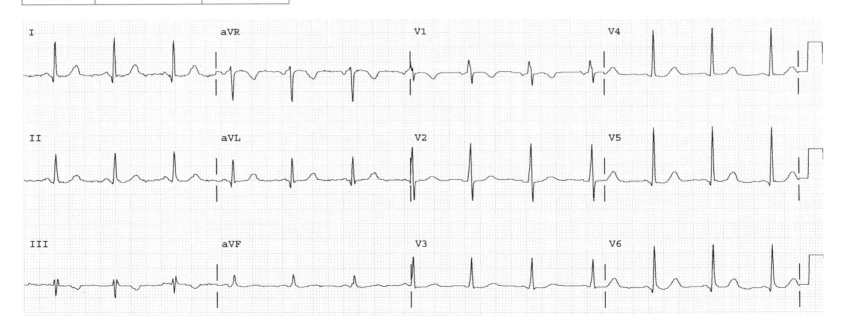

BASIC MEASUREMENTS			EVALUATION FOR ISCHEMIA OR INFARCTION		EVALUATION FOR SYSTEMIC EFFECTS: NOTE IF PRESENT	
Parameter	Measurement	Interpretation	T wave inversion		LAA/RAA/LVH/RVH	
HR			ST depression		Drug effect	
Rhythm			ST elevation		Hyper/ Hypokalemia	
PR			Q waves or equivalent		Hyper/ Hypocalcemia	
QRS					Low voltage	
QT					SI/QT III pattern	
QTc					Pericarditis	
P direction						
QRS direction						

A) Make basic measurements, evaluate for ischemia and infarction, and atrial abnormality.

B) Diagnose RVH if the QRS direction is either rightward, anterior, or both.

C) Evaluate clinically.

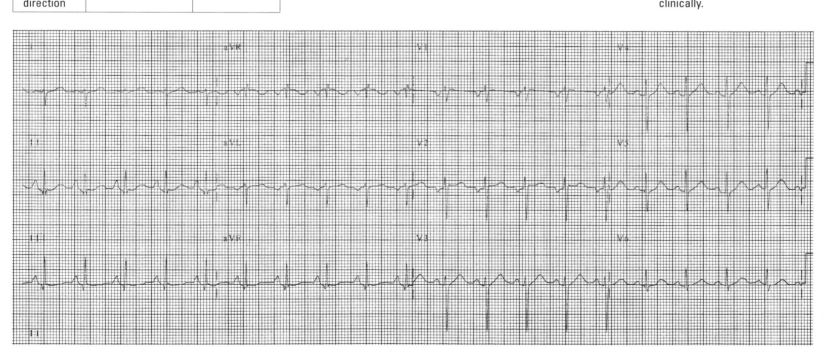

WORKSHEET VI.1

BASIC MEASUREMENTS			EVALUATION FOR ISCHEMIA OR INFARCTION		EVALUATION FOR SYSTEMIC EFFECTS: NOTE IF PRESENT	
Parameter	Measurement	Interpretation	T wave inversion		LAA/RAA/LVH/RVH	
HR			ST depression		Drug effect	
Rhythm			ST elevation		Hyper/ Hypokalemia	
PR			Q waves or equivalent		Hyper/ Hypocalcemia	
QRS						
QT					Low voltage	
QTc					SI/QT III pattern	
P direction					Pericarditis	
QRS direction						

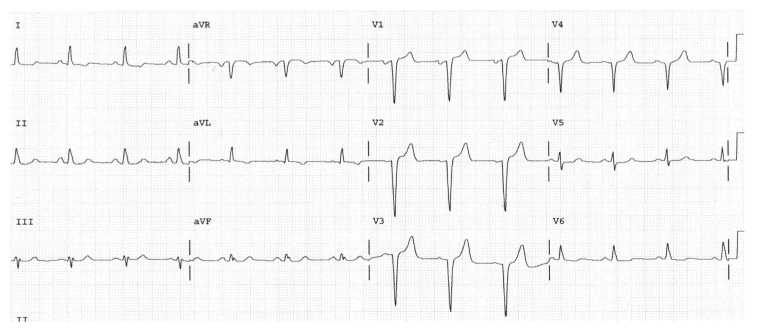

WORKSHEET VI.2

BASIC MEASUREMENTS			EVALUATION FOR ISCHEMIA OR INFARCTION		EVALUATION FOR SYSTEMIC EFFECTS: NOTE IF PRESENT	
Parameter	**Measurement**	**Interpretation**	T wave inversion		LAA/RAA/LVH/RVH	
HR			ST depression		Drug effect	
Rhythm			ST elevation		Hyper/ Hypokalemia	
PR			Q waves or equivalent			
QRS					Hyper/ Hypocalcemia	
QT					Low voltage	
QTc					SI/QT III pattern	
P direction					Pericarditis	
QRS direction						

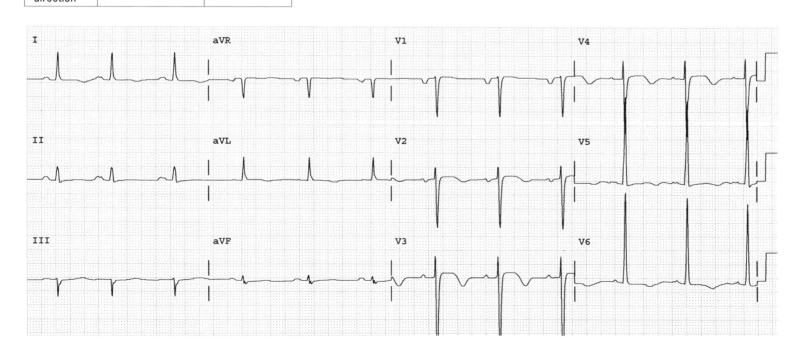

WORKSHEET VI.3

BASIC MEASUREMENTS			EVALUATION FOR ISCHEMIA OR INFARCTION		EVALUATION FOR SYSTEMIC EFFECTS: NOTE IF PRESENT	
Parameter	**Measurement**	**Interpretation**	T wave inversion		LAA/RAA/LVH/RVH	
HR			ST depression		Drug effect	
Rhythm			ST elevation		Hyper/ Hypokalemia	
PR			Q waves or equivalent			
QRS					Hyper/ Hypocalcemia	
QT					Low voltage	
QTc					SI/QT III pattern	
P direction					Pericarditis	
QRS direction						

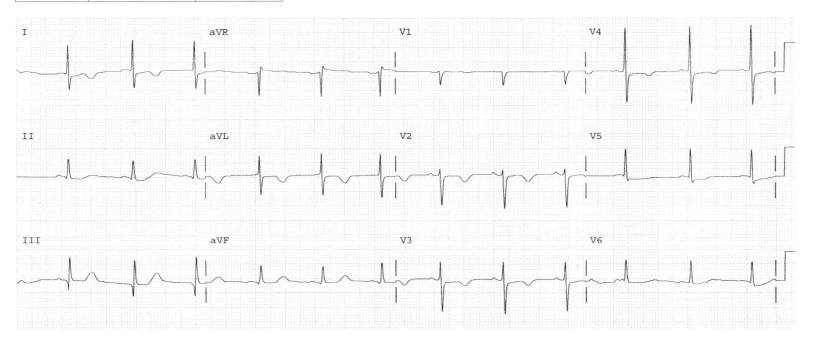

BASIC MEASUREMENTS			EVALUATION FOR ISCHEMIA OR INFARCTION		EVALUATION FOR SYSTEMIC EFFECTS: NOTE IF PRESENT	
Parameter	**Measurement**	**Interpretation**	T wave inversion		LAA/RAA/LVH/RVH	
HR			ST depression		Drug effect	
Rhythm			ST elevation		Hyper/ Hypokalemia	
PR			Q waves or equivalent			
QRS					Hyper/ Hypocalcemia	
QT					Low voltage	
QTc					SI/QT III pattern	
P direction					Pericarditis	
QRS direction						

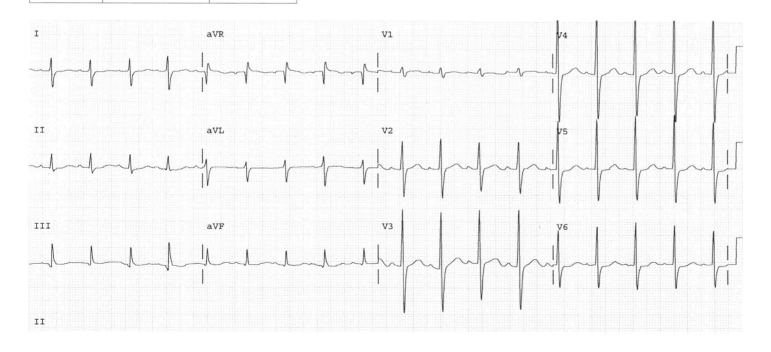

WORKSHEET VI.5

BASIC MEASUREMENTS			EVALUATION FOR ISCHEMIA OR INFARCTION		EVALUATION FOR SYSTEMIC EFFECTS: NOTE IF PRESENT	
Parameter	**Measurement**	**Interpretation**	T wave inversion		LAA/RAA/LVH/RVH	
HR			ST depression		Drug effect	
Rhythm			ST elevation		Hyper/ Hypokalemia	
PR			Q waves or equivalent		Hyper/ Hypocalcemia	
QRS					
QT					Low voltage	
QTc					SI/QT III pattern	
P direction					Pericarditis	
QRS direction						

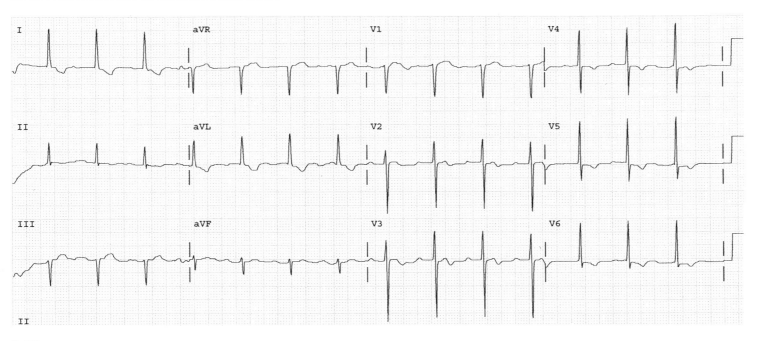

The Non-Ischemic Disorders: EKG Changes Related to Drugs, Electrolyte Abnormalities, and Other Diseases

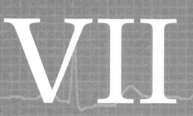

VII

Drug and Electrolyte Effects

Drug Effects: Digitalis

Digitalis is one of the oldest and most commonly used cardiac medications. In therapeutic doses, digitalis effectively slows the SA node from firing as often, slows conduction through the AV node, and increases contractility. When the blood levels of Digitalis exceed the therapeutic range, lethal dysrhythmia and EKG changes can occur. Digitalis toxicity produces various heart blocks, as well as ventricular dysrhythmias such as ventricular bigeminy and ventricular tachycardia. Digitalis toxicity produces a characteristic down sloping of the ST segment on the EKG. Figure 19.3 demonstrates junctional rhythm, a short QT interval, and diffuse "cheshire cat smile" ST depression in the inferior and lateral leads. The appearance of U waves in V2 represents coexisting hypokalemia, which exacerbates the digitalis effect.

Self-Study Objectives

■ **Define and identify EKG changes due to Drugs:**

Digitalis

Sotalol

Amiodarone

■ **Electrolytes abnormalities:**

Hyperkalemia

Hypokalemia

Hypercalcemia

Hypocalcemia

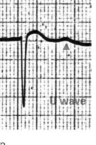

U wave

V2

FIGURE 19.1

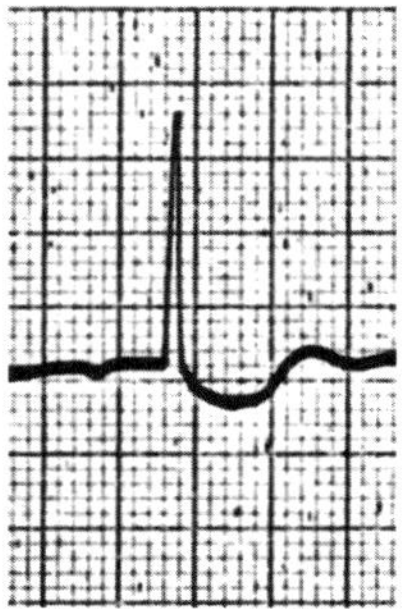

FIGURE 19.2

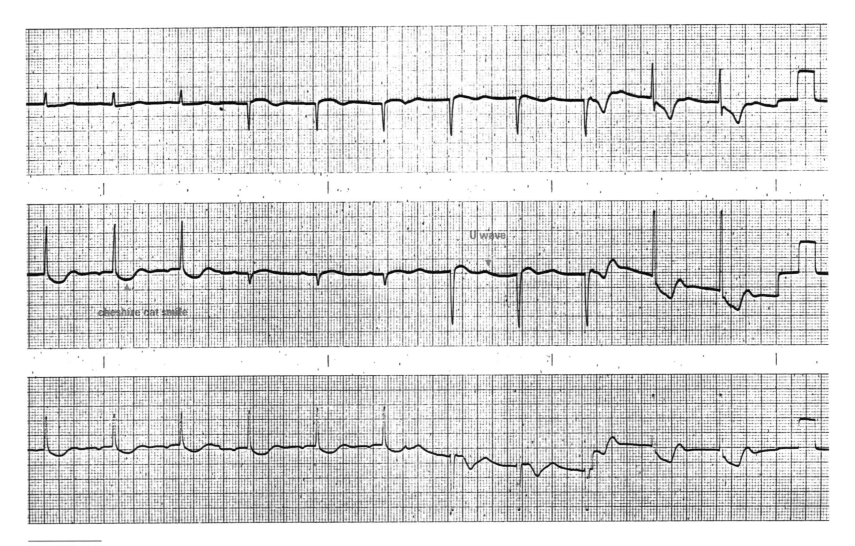

FIGURE 19.3

Drug Effects: Long QT Interval

Digitalis causes a short QT interval, but many drugs can be equally as dangerous by causing a long QTc interval. Common classes of these drugs are antiarrhythmics, antifungal agents, anaesthetics, antivirals, psychotropics, and chemotherapeutic agents. Figure 19.4a demonstrates a long QTc interval as a complication of Sotalol therapy, a Class III antiarrhythmic known to prolong the QTc interval. Amiodarone is another commonly used Class III antiarrhythmic which can have the same effect. Figure 19.4b demonstrates a visual reminder to help the reader double check the QTc. The normal T wave does not cross the midpoint between two QRS complexes.

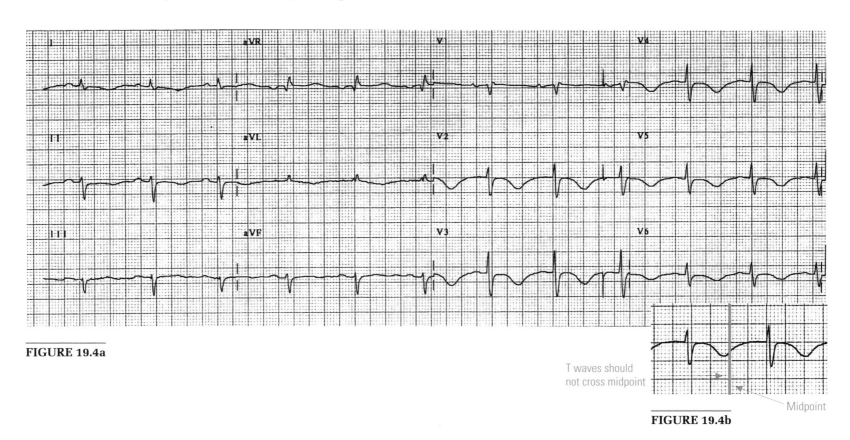

FIGURE 19.4a

T waves should not cross midpoint

Midpoint

FIGURE 19.4b

Electrolyte Effects: Hyperkalemia and Peaked T Waves

The normal electrical activity of the heart is dependent on the proper balance of specific serum electrolytes. Abnormal potassium (K+) levels have a direct effect on the normal electrical activity of the heart and of the myocardium. High serum potassium levels (hyperkalemia) depress conduction and impulse formation throughout the entire myocardium. This can initially produce peaked T waves on the EKG (Figure 19.5).

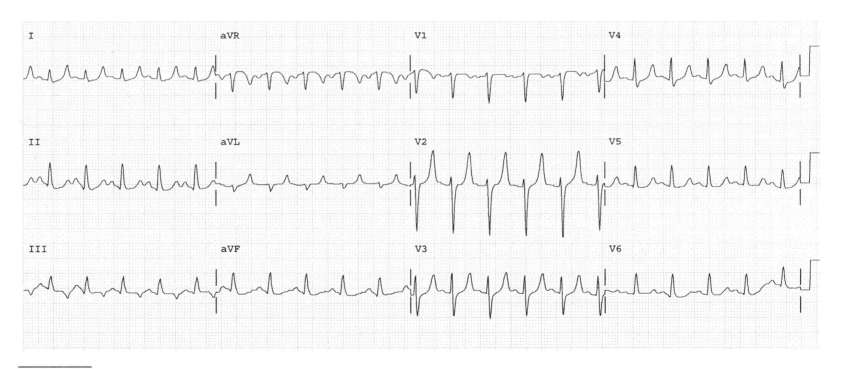

FIGURE 19.5

Electrolyte Effects: Hyperkalemia

Higher serum potassium levels, or hyperkalemia, depress conduction and impulse formation throughout the entire myocardium. This can result in drastic changes in the EKG. If the potassium level rise continues even higher or increases more acutely, a wide and bizarre looking sine wave-like pattern appears, as shown in Figure 19.6. (The patient's potassium level was 8.8 mEq/L when this was taken). Hyperkalemia is bizarrely wide (here 0.2 seconds) and doesn't have the same appearance as bundle branch block, which is usually 0.12 to 0.16 seconds wide. Furthermore, the rate is less than 100, so this is not ventricular tachycardia. If not immediately recognized and reversed, hyperkalemia eventually depresses the conduction system to the point of asystole and death. The standard emergency therapeutic regimen is the administration of glucose and insulin intravenously, which temporarily drives the potassium into the cells and out of the blood. Removal of the excess potassium from the body is done through the GI tract with an exchange resin (kayexalate), through the renal system with a diuretic, or by dialysis. A reader must immediately recognize and act on this EKG!

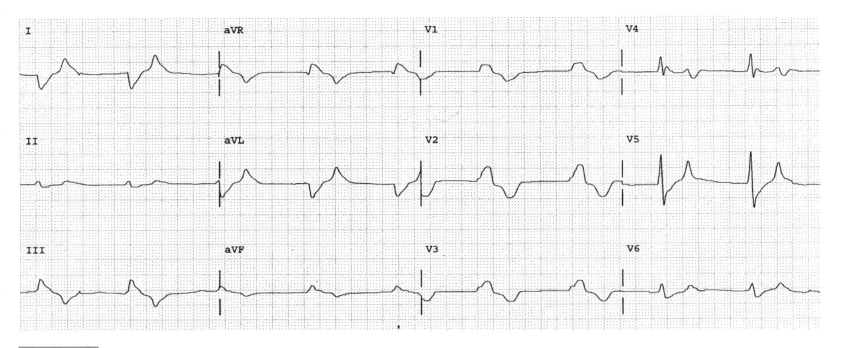

FIGURE 19.6a

Electrolyte Effects: Hyperkalemia Example of Progression and Reversal

Figure 19.6b demonstrates very wide QRS complexes that measure 0.20 seconds. This is not a typical bundle branch block because it is so wide. The T wave is tall wide and bizarre as well. Any QRS of 0.20 seconds suggests hyperkalemia until it is ruled out.

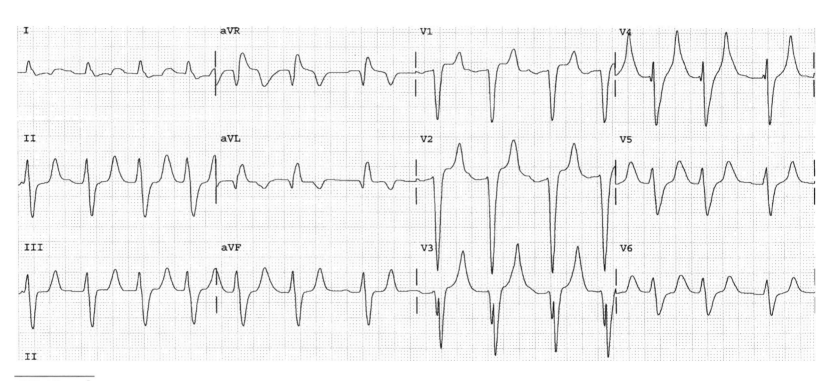

FIGURE 19.6b

Electrolyte Effects: Hyperkalemia Example of Progression and Reversal

Figure 19.6c was taken in the same patient as Figure 19.6b, but it was taken when the potassium level later rose to 9.8 mEq/Liter. The wide QRS complexes at the beginning of the strip may be confused with ventricular flutter, but the clear wide QRS complexes in V4 and V5 confirm the presence of hyperkalemia as the diagnosis. Recognition of Figure 19.b as hyperkalemia can help prevent the occurrence of Figure 19c.

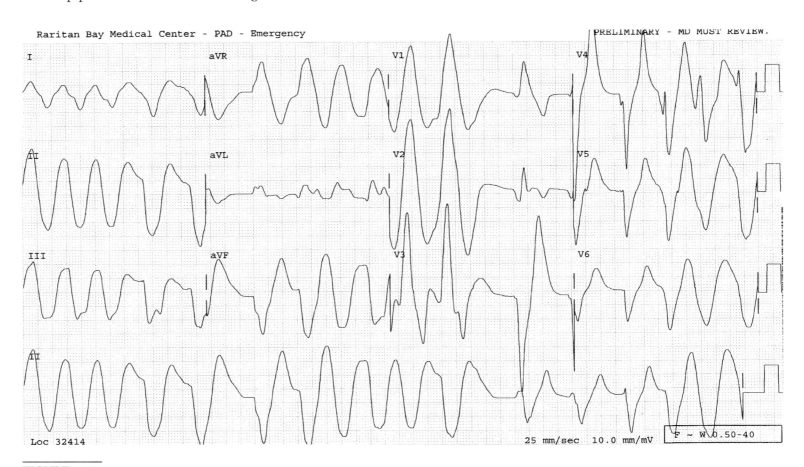

FIGURE 19.6c

Electrolyte Effects: Hyperkalemia Example of Progression and Reversal

Figure 19.6d demonstrates the normalization of the EKG to baseline for this patient after correction of the potassium level. The QRS now measures 0.11 seconds.

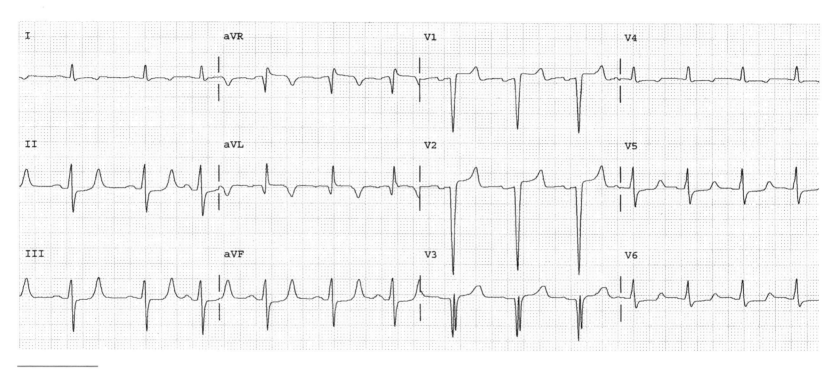

FIGURE 19.6d

Electrolyte Effects: Hypokalemia

A low serum potassium level, or hypokalemia, increases irritability of the conduction system and myocardium, thereby increasing the likelihood and frequency of ventricular ectopy. The increased irritability of the myocardium generates ventricular ectopic beats, PVCs, bigeminy, paired PVCs, ventricular tachycardia, and ventricular fibrillation. Hypokalemia produces flattened T waves. The QT interval becomes prolonged. *A low amplitude T wave due to hypokalemia is a common reason why the QT interval may be difficult to measure with confidence.* There can be diffuse ST segment depression, which looks like diffuse subendocardial ischemia (Figures 19.7, 19.8, 19.9). U waves (positive waves seen after the ST segment returns to baseline in the V leads) can sometimes be seen as well on the EKG. It is always clinically correct to worry about ischemia when ST depression or T wave inversion is present. It is essential to check the possibility of hypokalemia as well. The potassium level below was 1.7.

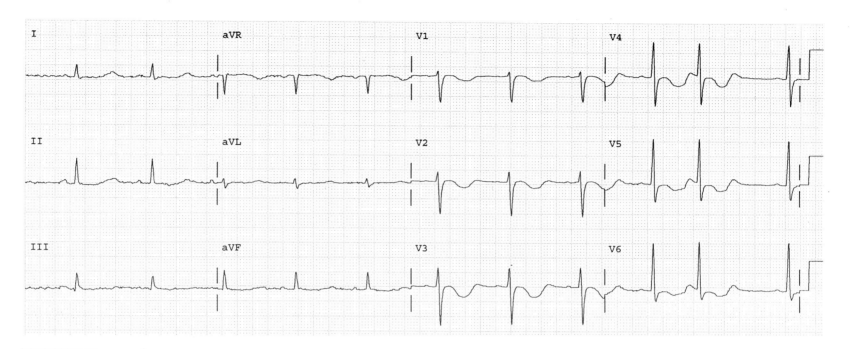

FIGURE 19.7

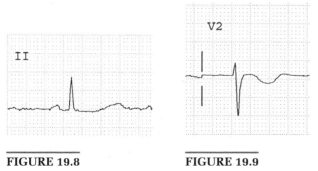

FIGURE 19.8

FIGURE 19.9

Electrolyte Effects: Hypercalcemia

A high serum calcium level (hypercalcemia) produces shortened QT intervals on the EKG. Hypercalcemia occurs in primary hyperparathyroididsm. It can also occur as a complication of metastatic cancer that has spread to bone. The mnenmonic Pb-Ktl (lead kettle) for prostate, breast, kidney, thyroid, and lung cancer, should raise the clinical possibility of bone metastases and possible hypercalcemia. The QT interval here (Figure 19.10) is 0.30 seconds. The QTc is 0.353 seconds. The serum calcium level was 12.8 in this patient. Even higher calcium levels can depress conduction and cause heart block.

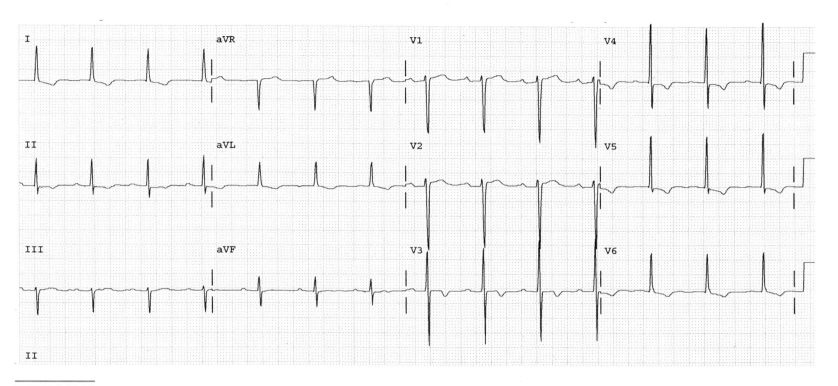

FIGURE 19.10

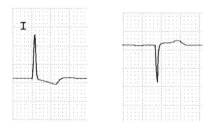

FIGURE 19.11   **FIGURE 19.12**

Electrolyte Effects: Hypocalcemia

Low serum calcium levels, or hypocalcemia, produce a prolonged QT interval (Figures 19.13, 19.14, 19.15). As with all casues of long QTc, ventricular tachycardia (torsade) or ventricular fibrillation can result. Clinically this can be seen in hypoparathyroidism and transfusion-related hypocalemia. Massive transfusion of packed red blood cells can cause hypocalcemia. Packed cells are poor in ionized calcium and contain a calcium binding agent to prevent clotting of the cells. The anticlotting agent in packed red cells binds to calcium. In Figure 19.13, the serum calcium level was 6.1. The QT measures 0.34 seconds, the QTc is 0.491.

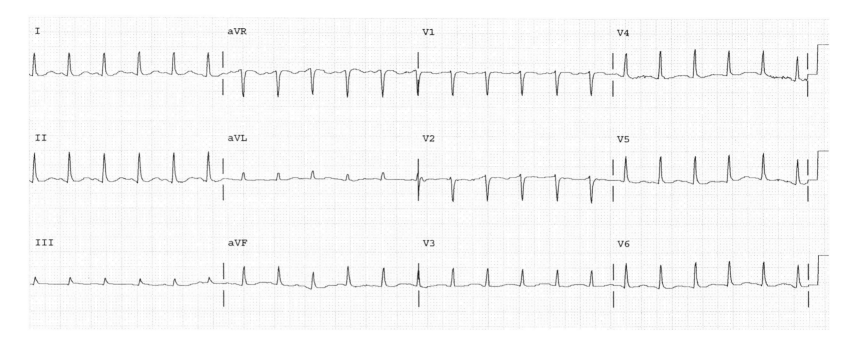

FIGURE 19.13

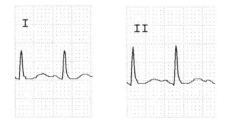

FIGURE 19.14   **FIGURE 19.15**

SAMPLE COMPLETED WORKSHEET

BASIC MEASUREMENTS

Parameter	Measurement	Interpretation
HR	56	Abnormal
Rhythm	Sinus Bradycardia	Abnormal
PR	0.16	Normal
QRS	0.08	Normal
QT	0.52	
QTc	0.502	Long
P direction		Normal
QRS direction		Normal

EVALUATION FOR ISCHEMIA OR INFARCTION

T wave inversion	Nonspecific inferior
ST depression	None
ST elevation	None
Q waves or equivalent	Nonspecific

EVALUATION FOR SYSTEMIC EFFECTS: NOTE IF PRESENT

LAA/RAA/LVH/RVH	
Drug effect	R/O
Hyper/Hypokalemia	R/O
Hyper/Hypocalcemia	R/O
Low voltage	
SI/QT III Pattern	
Pericarditis	

Instructions for Chapter 19 Worksheets

A) Make basic measurements, evaluate for ischemia and infarction, evaluate for hypertrophy.

B) Diagnose drug and electrolyte abnormalities as appropriate based on the heart rate, QRS, QTc and ST segments.

C) Evaluate clinically.

Clinically Based Critical Thinking: Interpretation

Sinus bradycardia is present. There is an abnormally long QTc. This suggests a drug toxicity or electrolyte abnormality. Antiarrhythmic therapy, hypokalemia, hypocalcemia, and so on should be considered and ruled out as causes. The offending agent should be removed if at all possible.

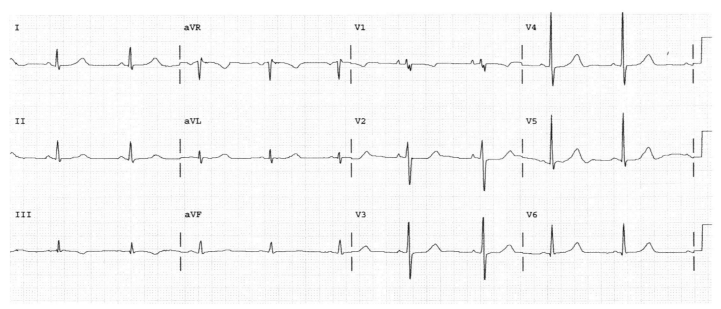

WORKSHEET 19.1

BASIC MEASUREMENTS			EVALUATION FOR ISCHEMIA OR INFARCTION		EVALUATION FOR SYSTEMIC EFFECTS: NOTE IF PRESENT	
Parameter	Measurement	Interpretation	T wave inversion		LAA/RAA/LVH/RVH	
HR			ST depression		Drug effect	
Rhythm			ST elevation		Hyper/ Hypokalemia	
PR			Q waves or equivalent			
QRS					Hyper/ Hypocalcemia	
QT						
QTc					Low voltage	
P direction					SI/QT III pattern	
QRS direction					Pericarditis	

Instructions for Chapter 19 Worksheets

A) Make basic measurements, evaluate for ischemia and infarction, evaluate for hypertrophy.

B) Diagnose drug and electrolyte abnormalities as appropriate based on the heart rate, QRS, QTc and ST segments.

C) Evaluate clinically.

Clinically Based Critical Thinking: Interpretation

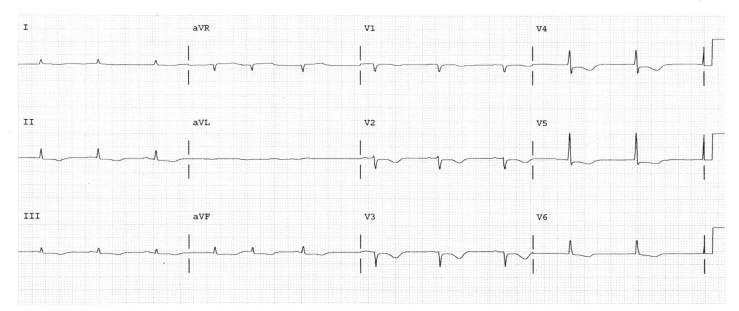

WORKSHEET 19.2

BASIC MEASUREMENTS			EVALUATION FOR ISCHEMIA OR INFARCTION		EVALUATION FOR SYSTEMIC EFFECTS: NOTE IF PRESENT	
Parameter	Measurement	Interpretation	T wave inversion		LAA/RAA/LVH/RVH	
HR			ST depression		Drug effect	
Rhythm			ST elevation		Hyper/ Hypokalemia	
PR			Q waves or equivalent			
QRS					Hyper/ Hypocalcemia	
QT						
QTc					Low voltage	
P direction					SI/QT III pattern	
QRS direction					Pericarditis	

Instructions for Chapter 19 Worksheets

A) Make basic measurements, evaluate for ischemia and infarction, evaluate for hypertrophy.
B) Diagnose drug and electrolyte abnormalities as appropriate based on the heart rate, QRS, QTc and ST segments.
C) Evaluate clinically.

Clinically Based Critical Thinking: Interpretation

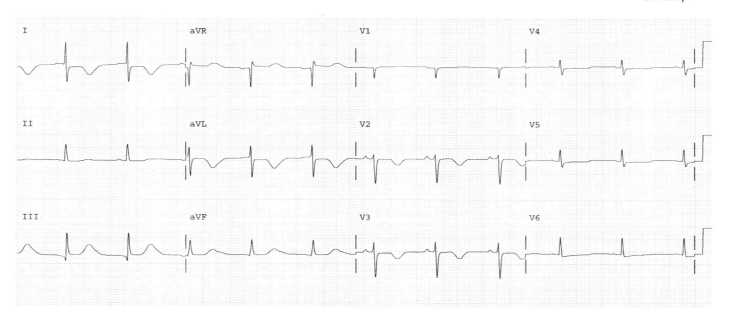

BASIC MEASUREMENTS			EVALUATION FOR ISCHEMIA OR INFARCTION		EVALUATION FOR SYSTEMIC EFFECTS: NOTE IF PRESENT	
Parameter	Measurement	Interpretation	T wave inversion		LAA/RAA/LVH/RVH	
HR			ST depression		Drug effect	
Rhythm			ST elevation		Hyper/ Hypokalemia	
PR			Q waves or equivalent		Hyper/ Hypocalcemia	
QRS					Low voltage	
QT					SI/QT III pattern	
QTc					Pericarditis	
P direction						
QRS direction						

Instructions for Chapter 19 Worksheets

A) Make basic measurements, evaluate for ischemia and infarction, evaluate for hypertrophy.

B) Diagnose drug and electrolyte abnormalities as appropriate based on the heart rate, QRS, QTc and ST segments.

C) Evaluate clinically.

Clinically Based Critical Thinking: Interpretation

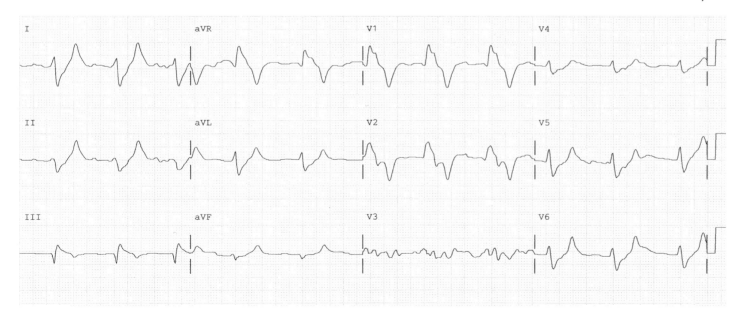

Clinical Conditions That Affect the EKG

--- Overview

The EKG not only provides valuable information on the electrical events of the heart, but it can also be useful in the diagnosis of medical and surgical conditions that affect the heart. Drug effects and toxicities, electrolyte imbalances, trauma, pericardial diseases, lung disease, cancer, cardiomyopathies, and systemic diseases are conditions that can cause specific changes on the electrocardiogram (Figure 20.1).

Self-Study Objectives

■ **Define and identify the associated EKG changes for:**

Pneumothorax

Pleural effusion

Dextrocardia

Pericardial effusion

Infiltrative cardiomyopathy

Pericarditis

Dilated cardiomyopathy

Hypertrophic cardiomyopathy

Chronic obstructive lung disease (COPD)

Athlete's heart

■ **Describe possible EKG changes associated with:**

Postoperative patients

Cancer patients

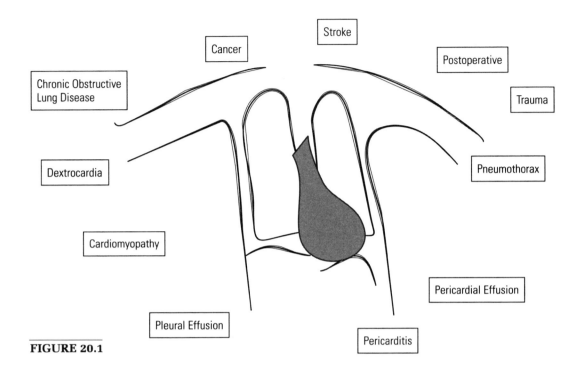

FIGURE 20.1

Low Voltage

The heart lies in the chest in the mediastinum, slightly to the left of the midline. There are certain diseases and conditions that alter the normal anatomy of the chest cavity and can cause changes in the EKG. When the changes in anatomy interfere with the ability of the EKG leads to take normal measurements, a condition called low voltage can occur (Figure 20.3). Low voltage is present in the frontal plane if the sum of the QRS amplitudes in leads I, II, and III (i.e., I + II + III) is less than 15 little boxes. Similarly, low voltage is present in the horizontal plane if the QRS amplitude does not reach 15 little boxes in at least one of leads V1, V2, or V3. Some examples of this are pneumothorax, large pleural effusion, obstructive lung disease, infiltrative cardiomyopathies, and dextrocardia.

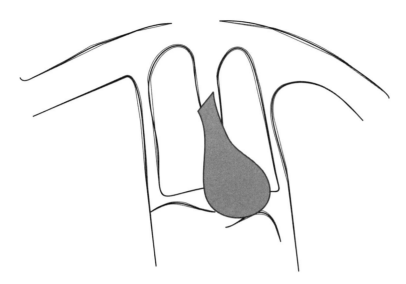

FIGURE 20.2

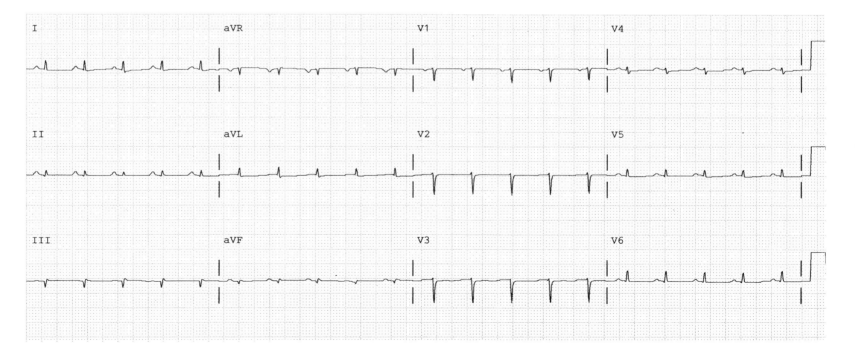

FIGURE 20.3

Low Voltage: Pneumothorax

A pneumothorax occurs when air seeps into the pleural space. The air interferes with the negative pressure in the pleural space and causes the lung to collapse. A pneumothorax can occur spontaneously (without any specific cause). It can also occur secondary to some form of chest trauma. The air in the pleural space pushes the heart away from the chest wall and, since air is a poor conductor of electricity, it makes the waveforms on the EKG smaller. Sinus tachycardia may be present and may indicate hemodynamic compromise or chest pain or anxiety.

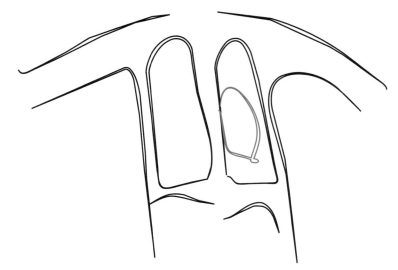

FIGURE 20.4

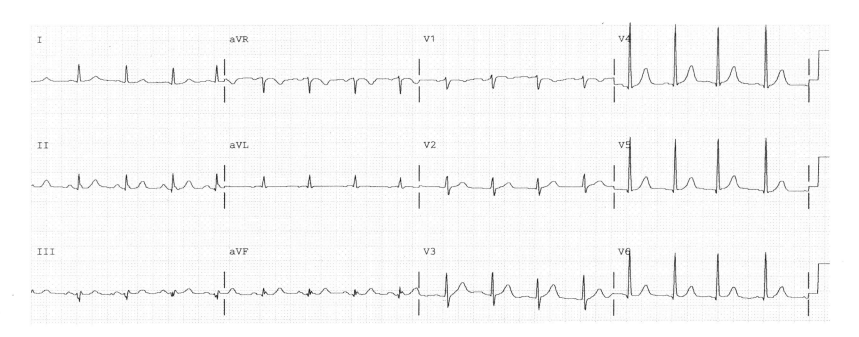

FIGURE 20.5

Low Voltage: Pleural Effusion

A pleural effusion is another condition that causes smaller wave-forms on the EKG. A pleural effusion is the term used for the build up of fluid in the pleural space. The build up of fluid in the pleural space is often associated with certain carcinomas, infection, congestive heart failure, or hemorrhage. In this instance, the fluid pushes the heart away from the chest wall and EKG leads. This is typically seen in a large left-sided pleural effusion.

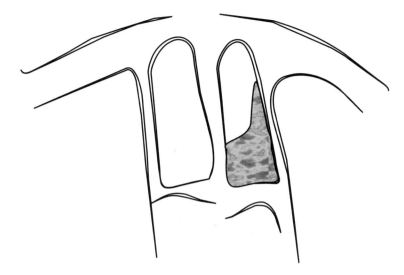

FIGURE 20.6

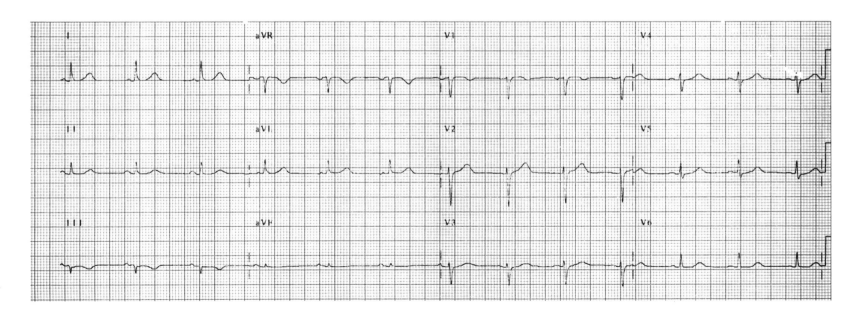

FIGURE 20.7

Low Voltage: Dextrocardia

Dextrocardia is another condition that may produce low voltage waves on the EKG. Dextrocardia is a congenital condition in which the heart is reversed in the frontal view in a mirror image of normal. Dextrocardia is a congenital defect that places the heart on the right side of the chest instead of the left side. This opposite position puts a greater distance between the heart and the precordial (chest) leads. The EKG shows decreased waveform voltages as the leads progress from lead V1 to V6. Since the leads were placed on the left side of the patient's chest, lead V2 is further from the heart than V1. V3 is further than V2, and so on. V6 is the furthest from the heart, and therefore has the lowest voltage of all. The P wave direction in the frontal plane points abnormally to the patient's right side (+135 degrees) and confirms the diagnosis.

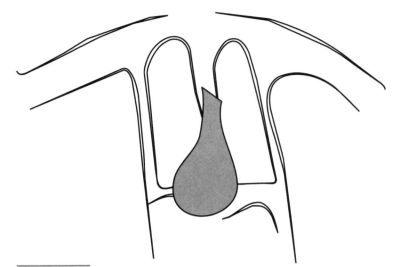

FIGURE 20.8

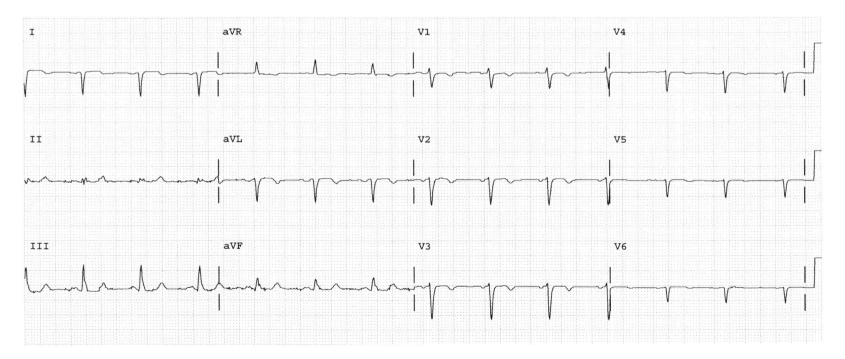

FIGURE 20.9

Low Voltage: Pericardial Effusion

A pericardial effusion is a condition in which the pericardial space fills with fluid, exudates, or blood. It is often the result of infection, trauma, carcinoma, hypothyroidism, or rheumatoid disease. The fluid in the pericardial space decreases the voltage that reaches the EKG leads, thereby producing smaller waveforms. Large or rapidly accumulating effusions can affect the hemodynamic status of the patient. Sinus tachycardia suggests hemodynamic compromise.

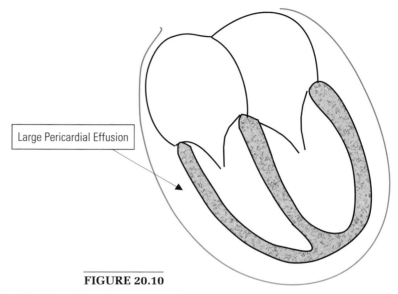

Large Pericardial Effusion

FIGURE 20.10

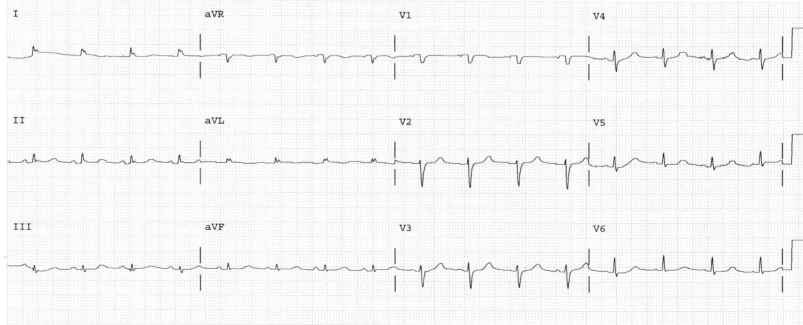

FIGURE 20.11

Low Voltage: Infiltrative Cardiomyopathy

Systemic diseases can affect the heart along with other parts of the body. Amyloid is a systemic disease that causes deposition of amyloid fibrils and casues thickening of the myocardium as measured by echo. Athough the myocardial walls appear thickened, EKG shows low voltage (Figure 20.12) because the thickened walls are not muscle but amyloid filler. The combination of low voltage on EKG and LVH on Echo (particularly in a speckled pattern) suggests amyloid disease of the heart.

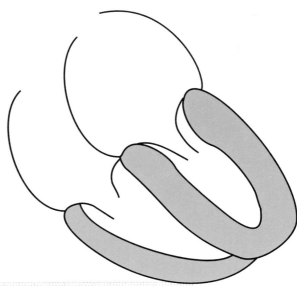

FIGURE 20.13

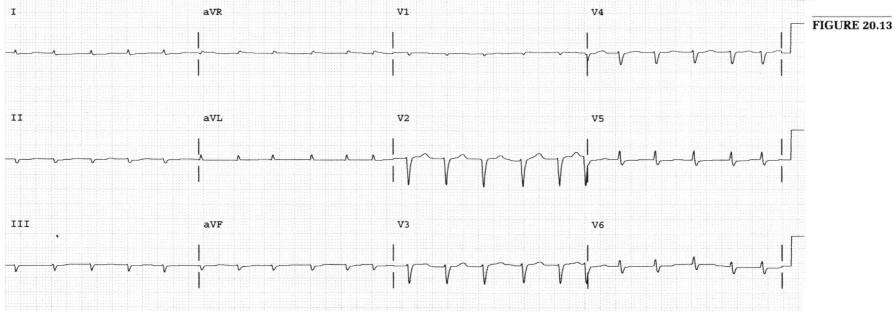

FIGURE 20.12

Pericarditis

Disorders of the pericardium can also produce specific changes in the EKG without causing a large collection of fluid and without causing low voltage. Pericarditis occurs when the pericardium becomes inflamed. Although the cause of pericarditis is not fully understood, it is associated with other disease processes, such as connective tissue disorders and infection. The inflammation of the pericardium can directly injure the underlying myocardium and mimic ischemia on the EKG. Sinus tachycardia may be present.

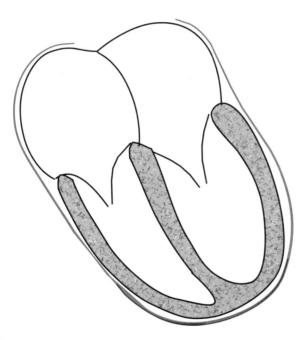

FIGURE 20.14

EKG in Pericarditis

Inflammation of the pericardium can cause changes on the electrocardiogram that can mimic ischemia or infarction. A rapid look at this EKG (Figure 20.15) could give the impression that the ST segment is elevated above the baseline in Lead II. An overly rapid interpretation of the EKG would describe the ST as elevated and pointing toward the inferior wall, consistent with transmural ischemia or infarction. However, after closer inspection, there is no ST segment elevation in the frontal plane. Rather it is an optical illusion caused by the presence of PT segment depression.

Now, look more carefully at the close-up of lead II, as shown here. The true baseline (arbitrarily, by definition) runs through the end of the T wave to the beginning of the P wave. There is no elevation of the ST segment in this lead. There is actually depression of the segment between the end of the P wave and the beginning of the QRS complex. This is PT segment depression, which is seen in pericarditis.

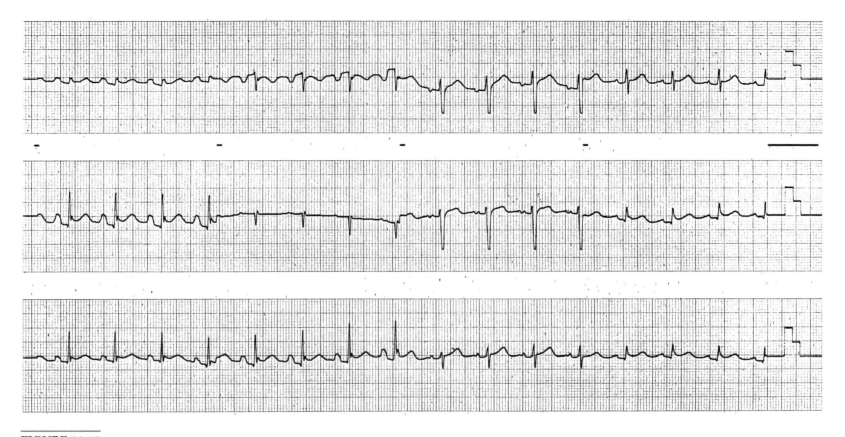

FIGURE 20.15

Now, look more carefully at the close-up of lead II, as shown here. The true baseline is shown in red and runs through the end of the T wave to the beginning of the P wave.

There is no elevation of the ST segment in this lead. This is an optical illusion. There is actually depression of the segment between the end of the P wave and the beginning of the QRS complex. This is PT segment depression, which is seen in pericarditis.

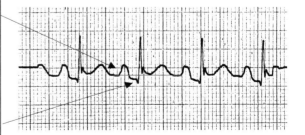

FIGURE 20.16

Dilated Cardiomyopathy

The EKG demonstrates abnormalities in many of the cardiomyopathies. Dilated cardiomyopathy is the diagnostic term used to describe a dilated and diffusely weakened heart muscle. Although in most cases the cause of cardiomyopathy is unknown, there are certain diseases, such as hypertension, viral infections, and alcoholism, that may contribute to it. The EKG may demonstrate left bundle branch block (Figure 20.18). Left atrial abnormality is another helpful clue.

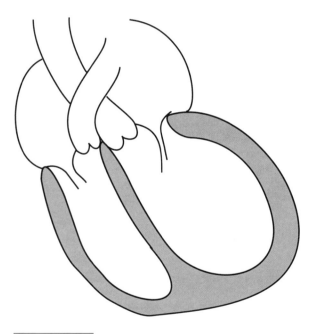

FIGURE 20.17

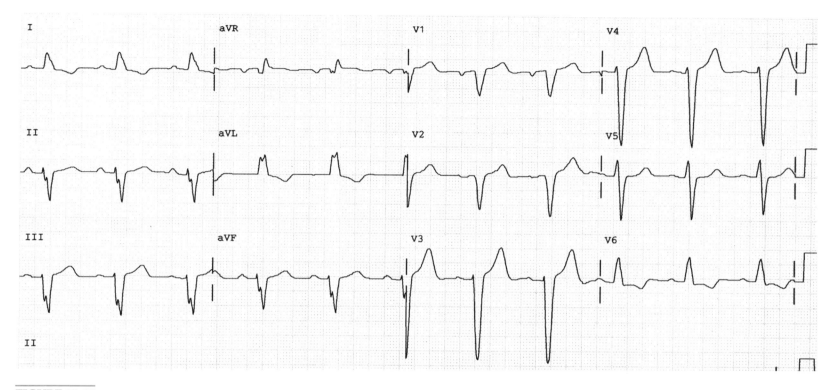

FIGURE 20.18

Hypertrophic Cardiomyopathy

Hypertrophic cardiomyopathy is associated with sudden death. This may include asymmetric hypertrophy of the ventricular septum, which produces increased voltage and criteria for left ventricular hypertrophy on the EKG. There may be dynamic outflow obstruction below the aortic valve as well. This is due to coaptation of the anterior mitral valve leaflet against the ventricular septum. This coaptation restricts the exit of blood from the left ventricle. This drop in cardiac output can cause syncope, shock, or sudden death. The EKG typically shows increased voltage but no obvious universal pattern of changes has been described. The presence of EKG evidence of LVH without a history of hypertension should prompt a workup for other causes of LVH.

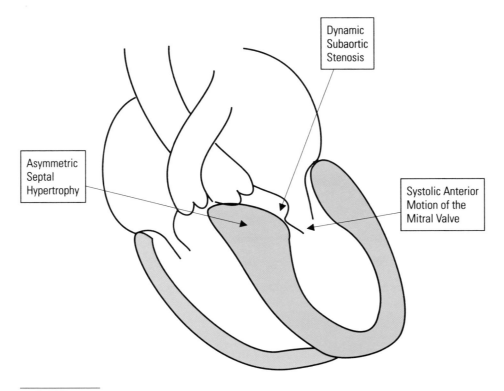

FIGURE 20.19

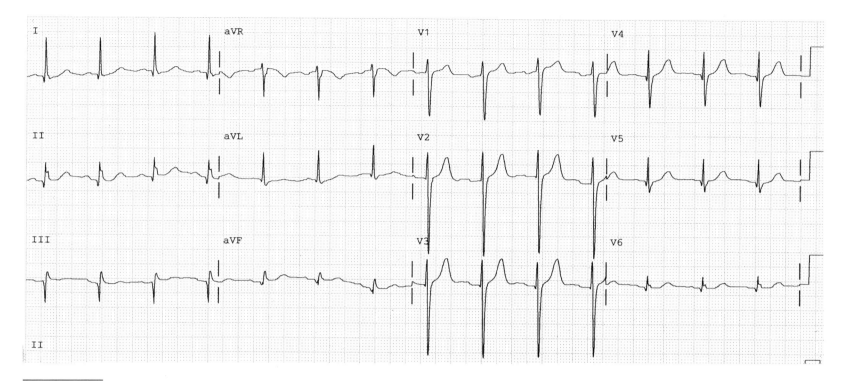

FIGURE 20.20

Chronic Lung Disease: Low Voltage

Chronic obstructive pulmonary disease (COPD) is a common disease and the most common cause of low voltage (Figure 20.22). Diseased airways trap excessive air in the lungs. Air is a poor conductor of electrical forces, and so the voltage of some or all leads on the EKG is lowered. Hypoxia or low oxygen level in the blood is another frequent cause of sinus tachycardia, when moderate or when the patient is treated with sympathetic agonists, or sinus bradycardia, when profound. All patients on ventilator support or those with chronic lung disease who develop sudden bradycardia should be evaluated immediately for hypoxia.

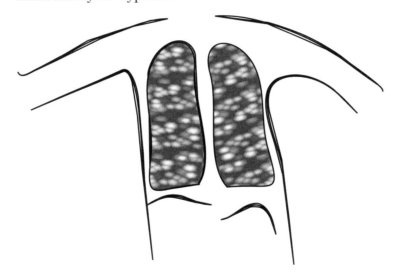

FIGURE 20.21

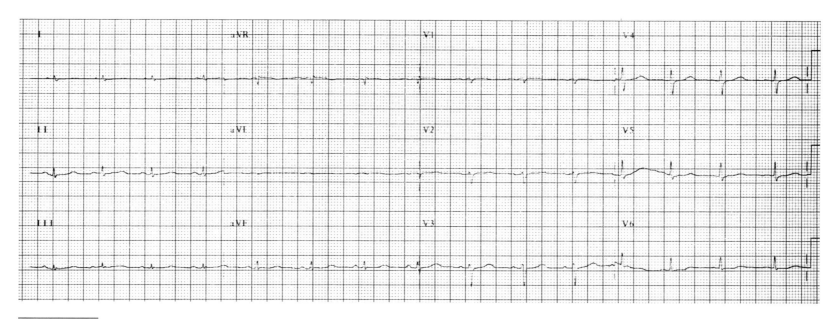

FIGURE 20.22

Athlete's Heart

The evaluation of the athlete's heart is always challenging for the clinician. Many of the EKG changes and dysrhythmias associated with an athlete's heart could represent a pathologic process in an average individual, but they are often considered normal for the well-conditioned person. Sinus bradycardia, sinus arrhythmia, sinus pause, escape beats, and various AV blocks are examples of dysrhythmias often experienced by an athlete. On the EKG, changes in the P wave and QRS complex are also common. Increased P wave voltage representing left or right atrial enlargement and increased QRS voltage representing right or left ventricular hypertrophy are often seen. Figure 20.23 demonstrates junctional rhythm and right intraventricular conduction delay (RSR in V1). Figure 20.24a demonstrates sinus arrhythmia. Figure 20.24b demonstrates 1° AV Block.

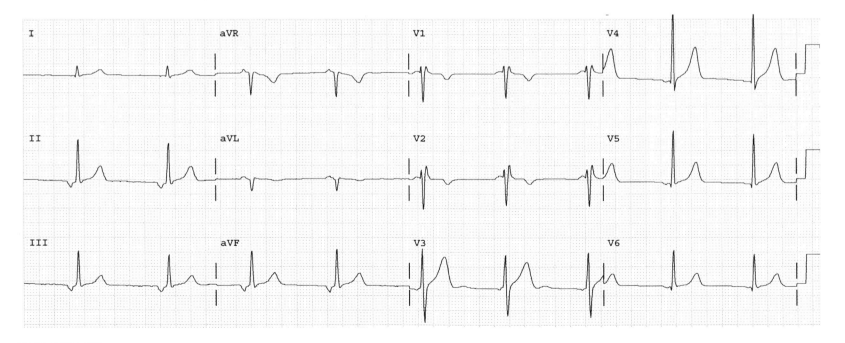

FIGURE 20.23

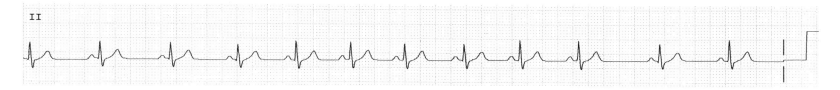

FIGURE 20.24a

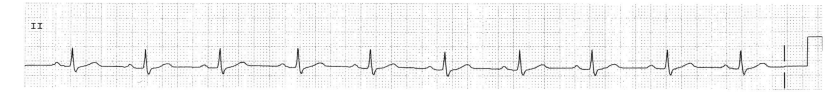

FIGURE 20.24b

Postoperative Patients: Sinus Tachycardia

When evaluating a patient with sinus tachycardia, the nurse or physician should assess the patient's level of pain. Pain stimulates the sympathetic nervous system, which causes the heart rate to rise. Postoperative patients who are experiencing pain and patients maintained on mechanical ventilators and not adequately sedated often develop sinus tachycardia. Once the patient is properly medicated and made comfortable, the heart rate often returns to normal. Other complications of surgery include pneumothorax, hypovolemia, and pulmonary embolism.

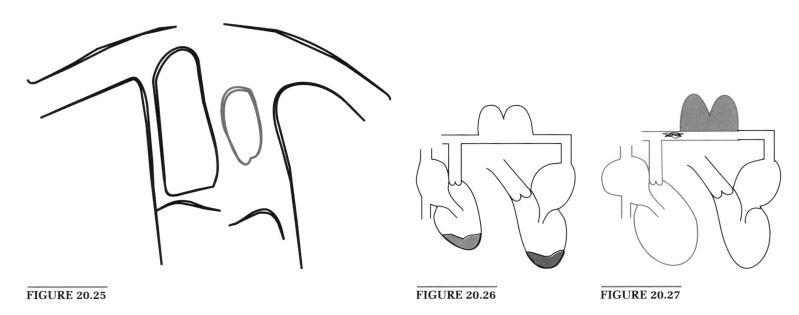

FIGURE 20.25   **FIGURE 20.26**   **FIGURE 20.27**

Effects of Cancer on the EKG

Malignant carcinomas and some cancer treatment modalities directly affect the heart and cause specific changes on the electrocardiogram. Pericardial effusion (Figure 20.28), tamponade, increased heart size, heart failure, and new heart murmurs are manifestations of malignant invasion of the heart. Radiation therapy can cause pericarditis. Chemotherapy can cause systolic heart failure, acutely or chronically. Hypercoagulable states can result in pulmonary embolism. Metastatic disease may also cause significant electrolyte disturbances. Obstructive or chemotherapy-induced renal failure may lead to hyperkalemia (Figure 20.29). Cancer patients may become hypovolemic (Figure 20.30) due to nausea and vomiting or bleeding. Metastatic spread to bone may be associated with hypercalcemia (Figure 20.31).

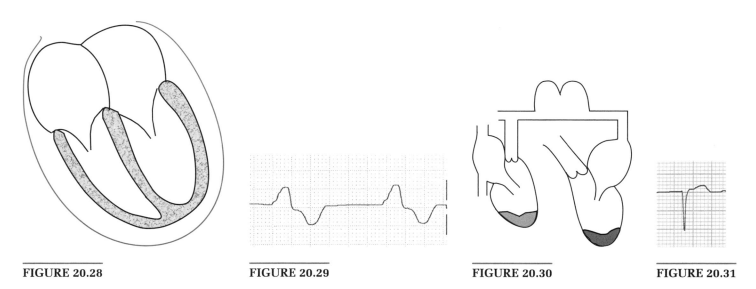

FIGURE 20.28   FIGURE 20.29   FIGURE 20.30   FIGURE 20.31

Effects of Stroke on the EKG

Subarachnoid hemorrhage has been classically associated with repolarization abnormalities on the EKG. Typical findings are deep symmetrically inverted T waves in the V leads, frequently associated with a long QT interval. Figure 20.32 demonstrates both of these. Possible drug and electrolyte causes of long QT, as well as cardiac ischemia or infarction, should also be considered.

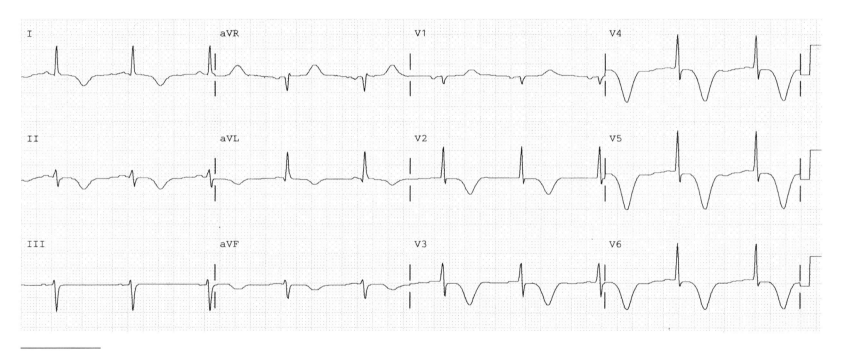

FIGURE 20.32

SAMPLE COMPLETED WORKSHEET

BASIC MEASUREMENTS			EVALUATION FOR ISCHEMIA OR INFARCTION		EVALUATION FOR SYSTEMIC EFFECTS: NOTE IF PRESENT	
Parameter	Measurement	Interpretation	T wave inversion	Nonspecific	LAA/RAA/LVH/RVH	
HR	115	Abnormal	ST depression	None	Drug effect	
Rhythm	Sinus tachycardia	Abnormal	ST elevation	None	Hyper/ Hypokalemia	
PR	0.12	Normal	Q waves or equivalent	Nonspecific	Hyper/ Hypocalcemia	
QRS	0.08	Normal			Low voltage	
QT	indeterminate				SI/QT III Pattern	
QTc					Pericarditis	
P direction		Normal				
QRS direction	anterior	RVH				

Instructions for Chapter 20 Worksheets

A) Make basic measurements, evaluate for ischemia and infarction, evaluate for hypertrophy.

B) Diagnose clinical conditions based on criteria described in Chapter 20.

C) Evaluate clinically.

Clinically Based Critical Thinking: Interpretation

There is sinus tachycardia associated with low voltage. Possibilities include COPD (with sinus tachycardia due to hypoxia or sympathomimetic therapy), or a large pericardial effusion or tamponade. The presence on an anterior QRS is consistent with pulmonary hypertension. The low amplitude affects the T waves and P waves as well.

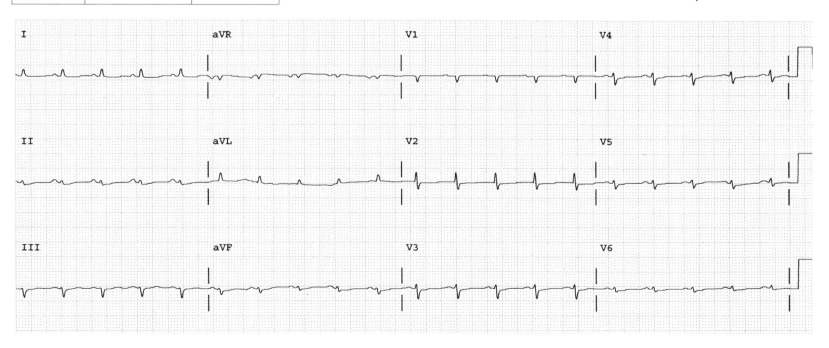

BASIC MEASUREMENTS			EVALUATION FOR ISCHEMIA OR INFARCTION		EVALUATION FOR SYSTEMIC EFFECTS: NOTE IF PRESENT	
Parameter	**Measurement**	**Interpretation**	T wave inversion		LAA/RAA/LVH/RVH	
HR			ST depression		Drug effect	
Rhythm			ST elevation		Hyper/ Hypokalemia	
PR			Q waves or equivalent		Hyper/ Hypocalcemia	
QRS						
QT					Low voltage	
QTc					SI/QT III pattern	
P direction					Pericarditis	
QRS direction						

Instructions for Chapter 20 Worksheets

A) Make basic measurements, evaluate for ischemia and infarction, evaluate for hypertrophy.
B) Diagnose clinical conditions based on criteria described in Chapter 20.
C) Evaluate clinically.

Clinically Based Critical Thinking: Interpretation

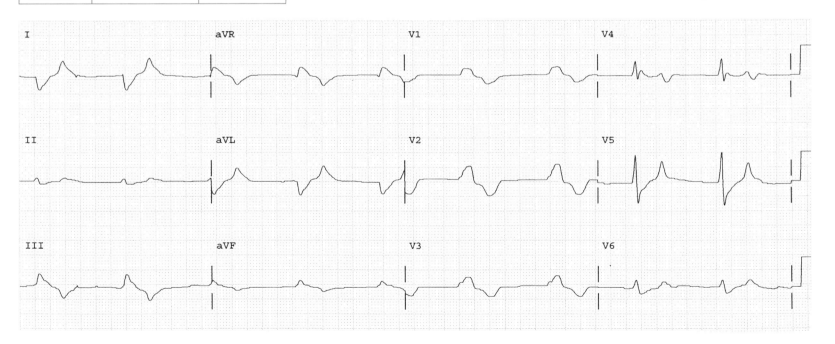

WORKSHEET 20.2

BASIC MEASUREMENTS			EVALUATION FOR ISCHEMIA OR INFARCTION		EVALUATION FOR SYSTEMIC EFFECTS: NOTE IF PRESENT	
Parameter	**Measurement**	**Interpretation**	T wave inversion		LAA/RAA/LVH/RVH	
HR			ST depression		Drug effect	
Rhythm			ST elevation		Hyper/ Hypokalemia	
PR			Q waves or equivalent		Hyper/ Hypocalcemia	
QRS						
QT					Low voltage	
QTc					SI/QT III pattern	
P direction					Pericarditis	
QRS direction						

Instructions for Chapter 20 Worksheets

A) Make basic measurements, evaluate for ischemia and infarction, evaluate for hypertrophy.
B) Diagnose clinical conditions based on criteria described in Chapter 20.
C) Evaluate clinically.

Clinically Based Critical Thinking: Interpretation

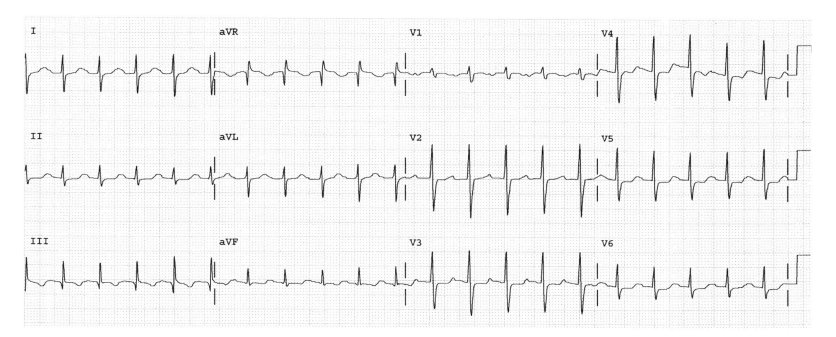

BASIC MEASUREMENTS			EVALUATION FOR ISCHEMIA OR INFARCTION		EVALUATION FOR SYSTEMIC EFFECTS: NOTE IF PRESENT	
Parameter	Measurement	Interpretation	T wave inversion		LAA/RAA/LVH/RVH	
HR			ST depression		Drug effect	
Rhythm			ST elevation		Hyper/ Hypokalemia	
PR			Q waves or equivalent			
QRS					Hyper/ Hypocalcemia	
QT					Low voltage	
QTc					SI/QT III pattern	
P direction					Pericarditis	
QRS direction						

A) Make basic measurements, evaluate for ischemia and infarction, evaluate for hypertrophy.

B) Diagnose clinical conditions based on criteria described in Chapter 20.

C) Evaluate clinically.

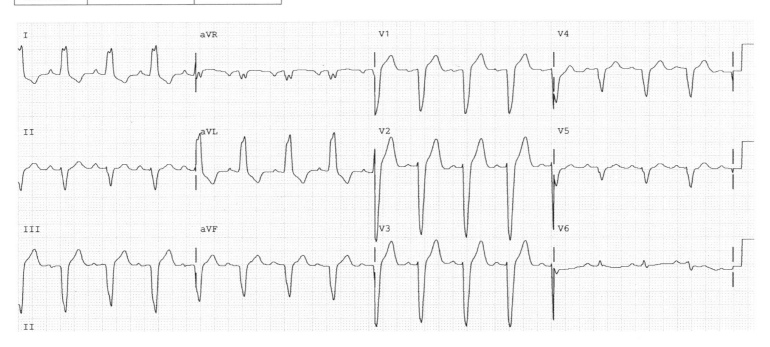

WORKSHEET VII.1

BASIC MEASUREMENTS			EVALUATION FOR ISCHEMIA OR INFARCTION		EVALUATION FOR SYSTEMIC EFFECTS: NOTE IF PRESENT	
Parameter	**Measurement**	**Interpretation**	T wave inversion		LAA/RAA/LVH/RVH	
HR			ST depression		Drug effect	
Rhythm			ST elevation		Hyper/ Hypokalemia	
PR			Q waves or equivalent		Hyper/ Hypocalcemia	
QRS					Low voltage	
QT					SI/QT III pattern	
QTc					Pericarditis	
P direction						
QRS direction						

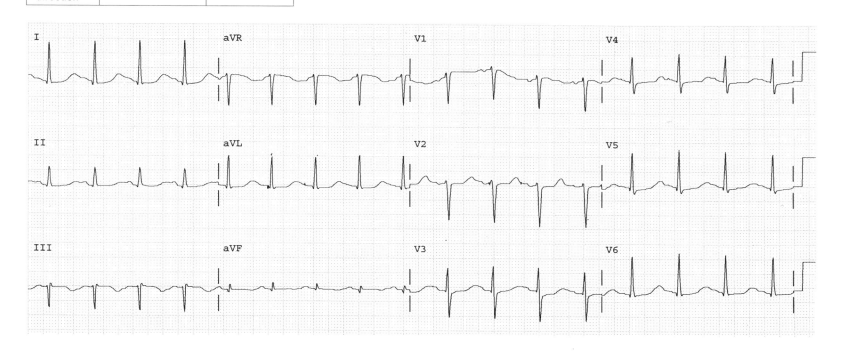

WORKSHEET VII.2

BASIC MEASUREMENTS			EVALUATION FOR ISCHEMIA OR INFARCTION		EVALUATION FOR SYSTEMIC EFFECTS: NOTE IF PRESENT	
Parameter	**Measurement**	**Interpretation**	T wave inversion		LAA/RAA/LVH/RVH	
HR			ST depression		Drug effect	
Rhythm			ST elevation		Hyper/ Hypokalemia	
PR			Q waves or equivalent		Hyper/ Hypocalcemia	
QRS						
QT					Low voltage	
QTc					SI/QT III pattern	
P direction					Pericarditis	
QRS direction						

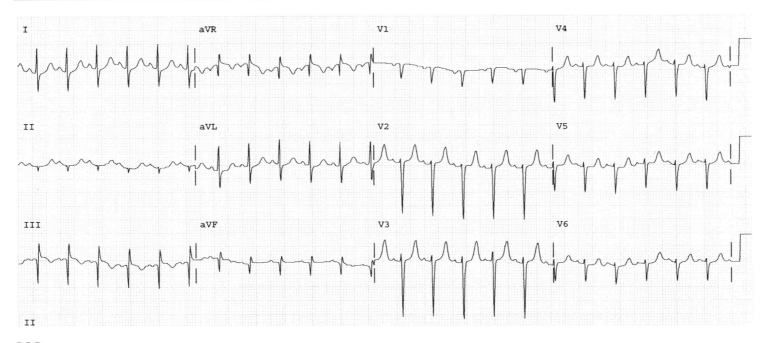

WORKSHEET VII.3

BASIC MEASUREMENTS			EVALUATION FOR ISCHEMIA OR INFARCTION		EVALUATION FOR SYSTEMIC EFFECTS: NOTE IF PRESENT	
Parameter	**Measurement**	**Interpretation**	T wave inversion		LAA/RAA/LVH/RVH	
HR			ST depression		Drug effect	
Rhythm			ST elevation		Hyper/ Hypokalemia	
PR			Q waves or equivalent			
QRS					Hyper/ Hypocalcemia	
QT					Low voltage	
QTc					SI/QT III pattern	
P direction					Pericarditis	
QRS direction						

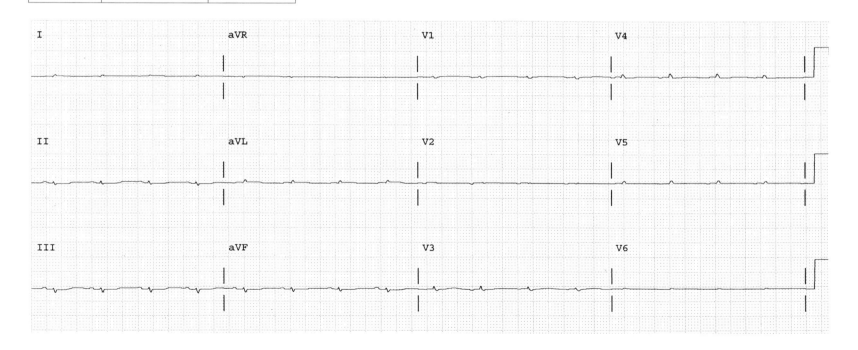

WORKSHEET VII.4

BASIC MEASUREMENTS			EVALUATION FOR ISCHEMIA OR INFARCTION		EVALUATION FOR SYSTEMIC EFFECTS: NOTE IF PRESENT	
Parameter	Measurement	Interpretation	T wave inversion		LAA/RAA/LVH/RVH	
HR			ST depression		Drug effect	
Rhythm			ST elevation		Hyper/ Hypokalemia	
PR			Q waves or equivalent			
QRS					Hyper/ Hypocalcemia	
QT					Low voltage	
QTc					SI/QT III pattern	
P direction					Pericarditis	
QRS direction						

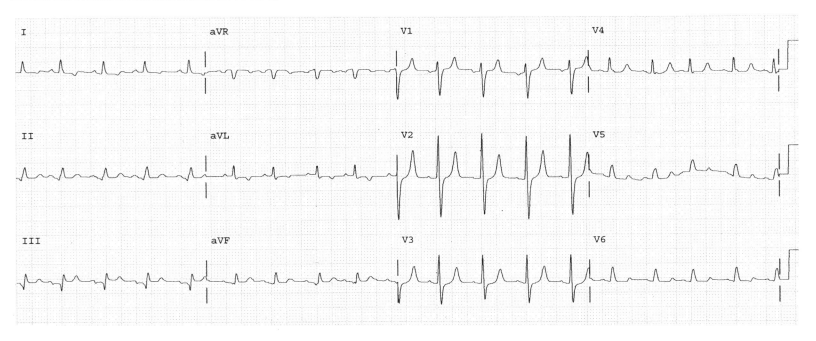

BASIC MEASUREMENTS			EVALUATION FOR ISCHEMIA OR INFARCTION		EVALUATION FOR SYSTEMIC EFFECTS: NOTE IF PRESENT	
Parameter	**Measurement**	**Interpretation**	T wave inversion		LAA/RAA/LVH/RVH	
HR			ST depression		Drug effect	
Rhythm			ST elevation		Hyper/ Hypokalemia	
PR			Q waves or equivalent		Hyper/ Hypocalcemia	
QRS						
QT					Low voltage	
QTc					SI/QT III pattern	
P direction					Pericarditis	
QRS direction						

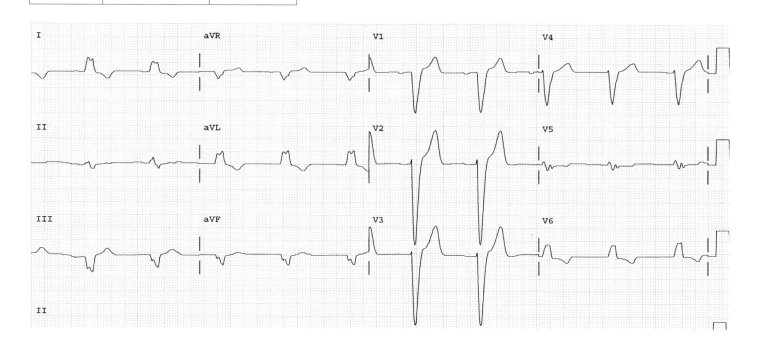

Self-Assessment

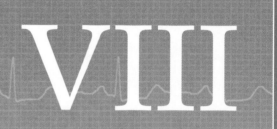

VIII

WORKSHEET VIII.1

Clinically Based Critical Thinking: Interpretation

BASIC MEASUREMENTS			EVALUATION FOR ISCHEMIA OR INFARCTION		EVALUATION FOR SYSTEMIC EFFECTS: NOTE IF PRESENT	
Parameter	**Measurement**	**Interpretation**	T wave inversion		LAA/RAA/LVH/RVH	
HR			ST depression		Drug effect	
Rhythm			ST elevation		Hyper/ Hypokalemia	
PR			Q waves or equivalent			
QRS					Hyper/ Hypocalcemia	
QT					Low voltage	
QTc					SI/QT III pattern	
P direction					Pericarditis	
QRS direction						

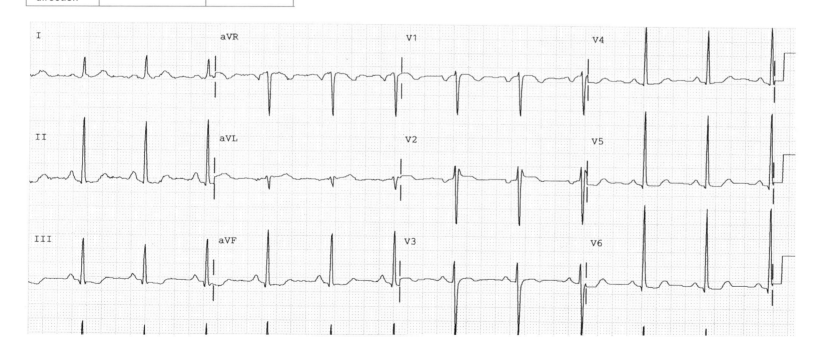

WORKSHEET VIII.2

BASIC MEASUREMENTS			EVALUATION FOR ISCHEMIA OR INFARCTION		EVALUATION FOR SYSTEMIC EFFECTS: NOTE IF PRESENT	
Parameter	Measurement	Interpretation	T wave inversion		LAA/RAA/LVH/RVH	
HR			ST depression		Drug effect	
Rhythm			ST elevation		Hyper/ Hypokalemia	
PR			Q waves or equivalent			
QRS					Hyper/ Hypocalcemia	
QT					Low voltage	
QTc					SI/QT III pattern	
P direction					Pericarditis	
QRS direction						

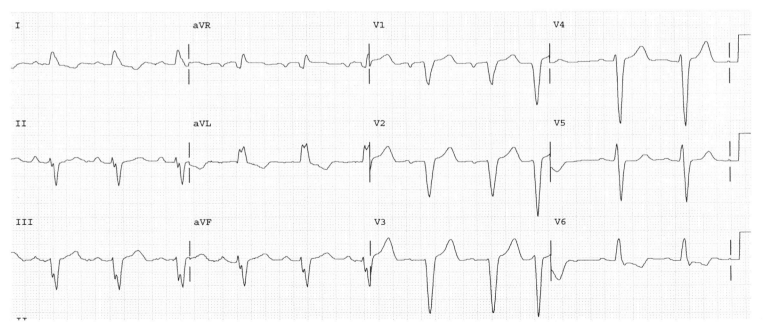

WORKSHEET VIII.3

BASIC MEASUREMENTS			EVALUATION FOR ISCHEMIA OR INFARCTION		EVALUATION FOR SYSTEMIC EFFECTS: NOTE IF PRESENT	
Parameter	**Measurement**	**Interpretation**	T wave inversion		LAA/RAA/LVH/RVH	
HR			ST depression		Drug effect	
Rhythm			ST elevation		Hyper/ Hypokalemia	
PR			Q waves or equivalent			
QRS					Hyper/ Hypocalcemia	
QT					Low voltage	
QTc		○			SI/QT III pattern	
P direction					Pericarditis	
QRS direction						

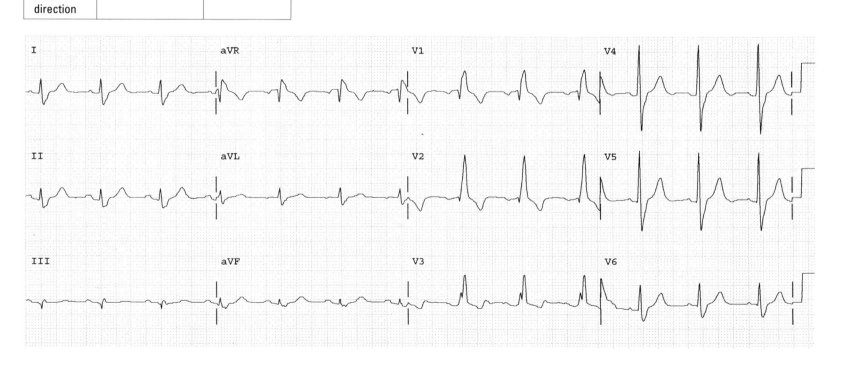

WORKSHEET VIII.4

BASIC MEASUREMENTS			EVALUATION FOR ISCHEMIA OR INFARCTION		EVALUATION FOR SYSTEMIC EFFECTS: NOTE IF PRESENT	
Parameter	Measurement	Interpretation	T wave inversion		LAA/RAA/LVH/RVH	
HR			ST depression		Drug effect	
Rhythm			ST elevation		Hyper/ Hypokalemia	
PR			Q waves or equivalent		Hyper/ Hypocalcemia	
QRS						
QT					Low voltage	
QTc					SI/QT III pattern	
P direction					Pericarditis	
QRS direction						

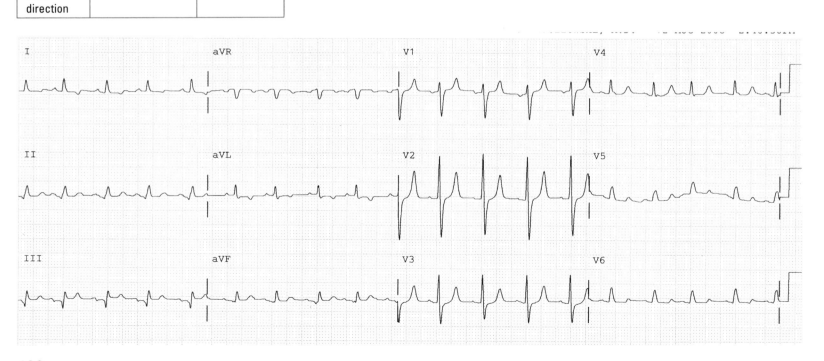

WORKSHEET VIII.5

BASIC MEASUREMENTS			EVALUATION FOR ISCHEMIA OR INFARCTION		EVALUATION FOR SYSTEMIC EFFECTS: NOTE IF PRESENT	
Parameter	**Measurement**	**Interpretation**	T wave inversion		LAA/RAA/LVH/RVH	
HR			ST depression		Drug effect	
Rhythm			ST elevation		Hyper/ Hypokalemia	
PR			Q waves or equivalent		Hyper/ Hypocalcemia	
QRS					Hyper/ Hypocalcemia	
QT					Low voltage	
QTc					SI/QT III pattern	
P direction					Pericarditis	
QRS direction						

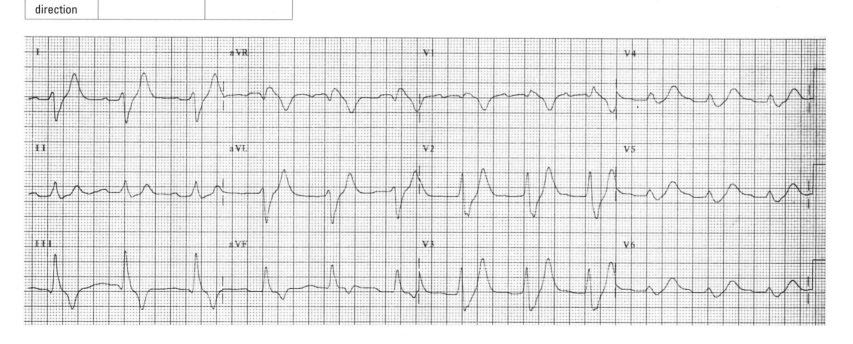

WORKSHEET VIII.6

BASIC MEASUREMENTS			EVALUATION FOR ISCHEMIA OR INFARCTION		EVALUATION FOR SYSTEMIC EFFECTS: NOTE IF PRESENT	
Parameter	**Measurement**	**Interpretation**	T wave inversion		LAA/RAA/LVH/RVH	
HR			ST depression		Drug effect	
Rhythm			ST elevation		Hyper/ Hypokalemia	
PR			Q waves or equivalent		Hyper/ Hypocalcemia	
QRS						
QT					Low voltage	
QTc					SI/QT III pattern	
P direction					Pericarditis	
QRS direction						

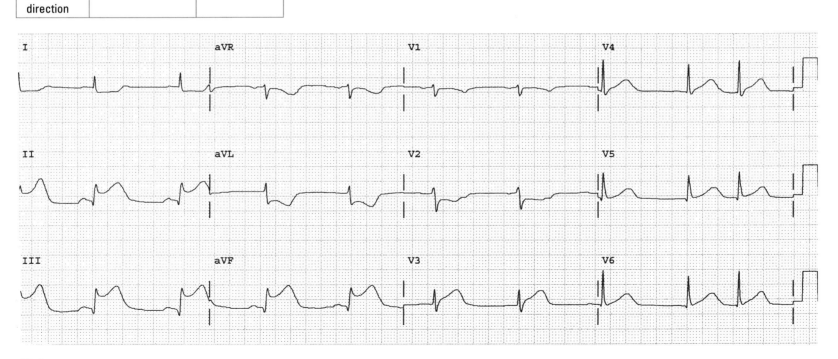

BASIC MEASUREMENTS			EVALUATION FOR ISCHEMIA OR INFARCTION		EVALUATION FOR SYSTEMIC EFFECTS: NOTE IF PRESENT	
Parameter	**Measurement**	**Interpretation**	T wave inversion		LAA/RAA/LVH/RVH	
HR			ST depression		Drug effect	
Rhythm			ST elevation		Hyper/ Hypokalemia	
PR			Q waves or equivalent		Hyper/ Hypocalcemia	
QRS					
QT					Low voltage	
QTc					SI/QT III pattern	
P direction					Pericarditis	
QRS direction						

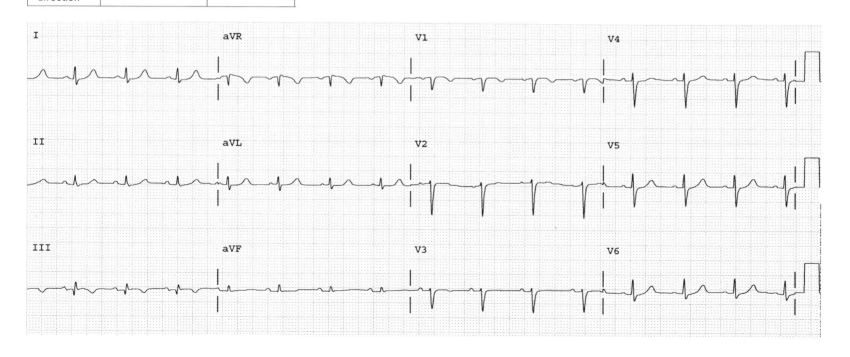

WORKSHEET VIII.8

BASIC MEASUREMENTS			EVALUATION FOR ISCHEMIA OR INFARCTION		EVALUATION FOR SYSTEMIC EFFECTS: NOTE IF PRESENT	
Parameter	Measurement	Interpretation	T wave inversion		LAA/RAA/LVH/RVH	
HR			ST depression		Drug effect	
Rhythm			ST elevation		Hyper/ Hypokalemia	
PR			Q waves or equivalent			
QRS					Hyper/ Hypocalcemia	
QT					Low voltage	
QTc					SI/QT III pattern	
P direction					Pericarditis	
QRS direction						

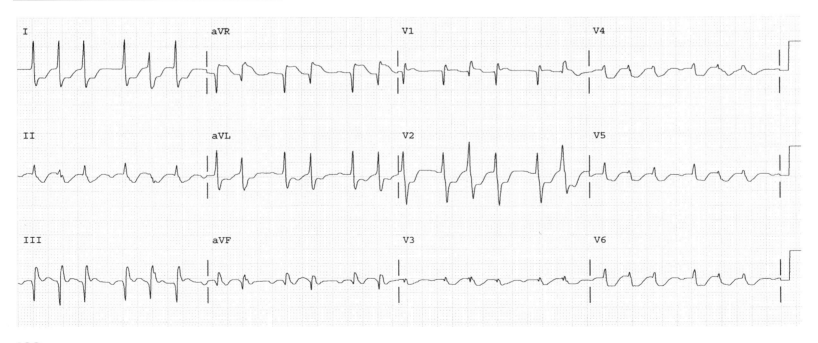

WORKSHEET VIII.9

BASIC MEASUREMENTS			EVALUATION FOR ISCHEMIA OR INFARCTION		EVALUATION FOR SYSTEMIC EFFECTS: NOTE IF PRESENT	
Parameter	Measurement	Interpretation	T wave inversion		LAA/RAA/LVH/RVH	
HR			ST depression		Drug effect	
Rhythm			ST elevation		Hyper/ Hypokalemia	
PR			Q waves or equivalent		Hyper/ Hypocalcemia	
QRS					Low voltage	
QT					SI/QT III pattern	
QTc					Pericarditis	
P direction						
QRS direction						

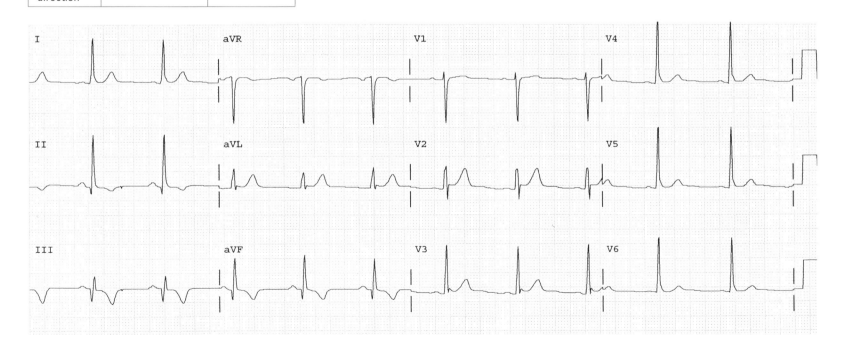

WORKSHEET VIII.10

BASIC MEASUREMENTS			EVALUATION FOR ISCHEMIA OR INFARCTION		EVALUATION FOR SYSTEMIC EFFECTS: NOTE IF PRESENT	
Parameter	**Measurement**	**Interpretation**	T wave inversion		LAA/RAA/LVH/RVH	
HR			ST depression		Drug effect	
Rhythm			ST elevation		Hyper/ Hypokalemia	
PR			Q waves or equivalent		Hyper/ Hypocalcemia	
QRS						
QT					Low voltage	
QTc					SI/QT III pattern	
P direction					Pericarditis	
QRS direction						

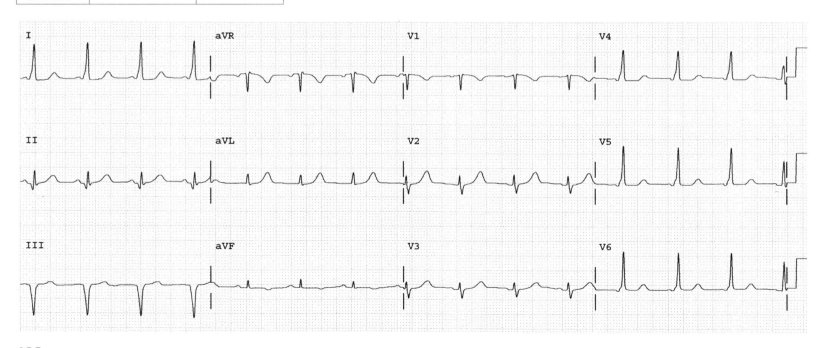

ANSWERS TO EKG WORKSHEETS

Section II

Chapter 4

4.1 The HR is 83 bpm. The rhythm is sinus. Sinus rhythm indicates relative balance between sympathetic and parasympathetic effects on the heart.

4.2 The HR is 125. The rhythm is sinus tachycardia. Sinus tachycardia indicates sympathetic predominance. Shock, heart failure, sepsis, hyperthyroidism, and hypovolemia should be considered.

4.3 The HR is 50. The rhythm is sinus bradycardia. The fourth and seventh beats are nonspecific PACs. The presence of sinus bradycardia indicates relative inhibition of the sympathetic nervous system. Most commonly this is due to medications such as beta blockers.

Chapter 5

5.1 The HR is 60. This is sinus rhythm. The PR interval is 0.18 to 0.20 seconds and is normal. The QRS interval is 0.10 seconds long, consistent with intraventricular conduction delay (IVCD). The QT interval is 0.40 seconds. The calculated QTc is 0.40, which is normal.

5.2 The HR is 71 bpm. This is sinus rhythm. The PR interval is 0.16 seconds and is normal. The QRS interval is 0.12 seconds (in leads I and AVL) and indicates bundle branch block. The QT interval is 0.40 seconds. The calculated QTc is 0.435 which

is normal. The clinical significance of bundle branch block is discussed in Chapters 11 and 12.

5.3 The HR is 88 bpm. The rhythm is sinus. The PR interval is 0.18 and is normal. The QRS interval is 0.14 seconds and is abnormal. This indicates bundle branch block. The QT interval is 0.40 seconds. The calculated QTc is 0.48 which is abnormal and long. Possibilities include drug effects such as sotalol, amiodarone, macrolide antibiotics, antifungal agents, and psychotropics, as well as hypokalemia and hypocalcemia.

Chapter 6

6.1 The HR is 75. This is sinus rhythm. The PR is 0.12 seconds, normal. The QRS is 0.08 seconds, and normal. The QT is 0.36 seconds. The QTc is normal. The P direction is inferior and leftward which is normal. The normal P axis confirms that the EKG was taken correctly, and may be interpreted normally.

6.2 The HR is 65. The P direction is very abnormal and points upward (it's negative in AVF) and to the patient's right side (it's negative in lead I). Possibilities for an upward pointing P wave include junctional rhythm. Possibilities for a rightward P include dextrocardia and arm lead misplacement. The patient should be examined, and a repeat EKG done carefully to determine which diagnosis is correct.

6.3 The HR is 71 bpm and is normal. The P axis is abnormal. It is negative in lead I, so it is pointing to the patient's right side. This indicates dextrocardia or arm lead misplacement. The patient should be examined and a repeat EKG done carefully to determine which is correct.

Section II Worksheets

II.1 The HR is 54. This is sinus bradycardia and indicates relatively decreased sympathetic tone. The PR interval is 0.28 seconds which is long and indicates 1° AVB. The QRS interval is 0.08 seconds and normal. The QT interval is 0.52 seconds or more. The calculated QTc is 0.493 which is long and should always suggest the possibility of a drug or electrolyte problem. The P direction is normal.

II.2 The HR is 75, the rhythm is sinus. The PR interval is too short, and a slurred upstroke is seen at the beginning of the QRS in leads 1 and AVL as well as in V1 through V6. This is WPW.

II.3 The HR is 83 bpm, the rhythm is sinus. The PR is 0.12 to 0.14 and normal. The QRS interval is 0.14 seconds, and long. This is bundle branch block. The QT interval is 0.40 seconds. The QTc calculates to 470 which is long. The P direction is normal.

II.4 The HR is 71 bpm. The rhythm is sinus. The PR interval is 0.16 seconds and normal. The QRS interval is 0.08 seconds and normal. The T wave is barely visible in the limb leads and so the QT interval is indeterminate. This suggests a drug or electrolyte problem, frequently hypokalemia. The P direction is leftward, but cannot be seen in lead AVF.

II.5 The HR is 83 bpm. The rhythm is sinus. The PR interval is 0.14 seconds and normal. The QRS interval is 0.08 seconds and normal. The QT interval is 0.42. The calculated QTc is 0.49 which is long. The patient's K^+ was 2.8 mEq/Liter. The P direction is normal.

Section III

Chapter 7

7.1 Atrial flutter.
7.2 Arrhythmia. Rate varies from 60 to 75.
7.3 Atrial fibrillation. Ventricular rate 180.

Chapter 8

8.1 Ventricular fibrillation
8.2 Polymorphous ventricular tachycardia (Torsade)
8.3 Artifact. This is a dual channel recording. Note the bottom strip shows the patient in sinus rhythm.

Chapter 9

9.1 2nd degree AV block (2° AVB) Type I, Wenckebach, with 4 to 3 conduction. The PR interval gradually increases until a QRS is dropped. There are 4 P waves to 3 QRS complexes, thus a 4 to 3 ratio.

9.2 Atrial pacing. A discrete vertical spike of a pacing artifact is present 0.28 seconds before the QRS.

9.3 The top strip shows ventricular pacing and a long QTc. The bottom strip taken later shows torsade.

Section III Worksheets

III.1 Sinus rhythm.
III.2 1° degree AV block.
III.3 Sinus rhythm with two PAC's.
III.4 CHB, atrial rate 79, ventricular rate 37.
III.5 PVC, followed by 3:2 and 2:1 Wenckebach.
III.6 Sinus rhythm with two PAC's.
III.7 Ventricular tachycardia.
III.8 Asystole.
III.9 Atrial and ventricular pacing. The pacing spike hits the T wave, causing V Tach, and V fib.
III.10 Atrial flutter with 6:1 conduction.
III.11 PVC.
III.12 1°AV block, 2:1 2°AVB.
III.13 Atrial fibrillation, ventricular rate 180.
III.14 Sinus rhythm with first degree AV block, and a PAC.
III.15 2 dropped P waves. 2°AV block, Type II.

Section IV

Chapter 10

10.1 HR 65. Sinus rhythm. PR 0.12 to 0.14, normal. QRS 0.12, bundle branch block. The QT is 0.44. The P direction is normal. The QRS direction is upward at −45°, since it is negative in leads II, III, and AVF. This is LAHB.

10.2 HR 107. Rhythm sinus tachycardia. PR 0.16. The QRS is 0.12 seconds, consistent with bundle branch block. The QT is 0.36. The P direction is normal. The QRS direction is rightward since it is overall negative in lead I. There is much more area in the S wave than the R wave in lead I, so the QRS is considered negative. This is LPHB.

10.3 HR 107. Sinus tachycardia. PR 0.12, normal. QRS 0.11, IVCD. The QT is 0.32. The P direction is normal. The QRS direction is abnormal and points upward since it is negative in leads II, III, and AVF. This is LAHB.

Chapter 11

11.1 HR 75, sinus. The PR is 0.16, normal. The QRS is 0.12 seconds indicating bundle branch block. The end of the QRS is negative in lead I, and so points to the right ventricle. The end of the QRS is positive in lead V1 and so points to the right ventricle. Therefore there is RBBB. The P direction is normal. The QRS overall direction is normal, so hemiblock is not present.

11.2 HR 65, sinus rhythm. The PR is 0.16, normal. The QRS is 0.12 seconds indicating bundle branch block. The end of the QRS is negative in lead I, pointing to the right. The end of the QRS is positive in lead V1 pointing to the right ventricle as well. This is RBBB. The P direction is normal. The overall QRS direction is rightward, since the area under the curve for the S wave is more than the R wave. This is LPHB.

11.3 HR 103. Sinus tachycardia. A PAC is seen in lead V1. The PR is 0.12, normal. The QRS interval is 0.13, indicating bundle

branch block. The end of the QRS is negative in lead I (so pointing to the right), and positive in lead V1 (so pointing anterior). This is RBBB. The QT is 0.32. The P direction is normal. The overall QRS direction is rightward, since lead I is negative. This is LPHB. Sinus tachycardia indicates sympathetic stimulation.

Chapter 12

12.1 Rate 115, sinus tachycardia. PR 0.12, normal. QRS 0.12 BBB. The end of the QRS is positive in lead I and so points to the left ventricle. The end of the QRS is negative in lead V1, and so points posteriorly and to the left ventricle as well. This is LBBB. The QT interval is 0.32. The QTc is 0.44.

12.2 Wide QRS tachycardia at rate of 124. The P waves are not clearly visible. This may represent sinus tachycardia with LBBB. It may also represent ventricular tachycardia.

12.3 HR 75, sinus rhythm. The QRS is 0.16 seconds, BBB. The end of the QRS is positive in lead I, and negative in lead V1 pointing to the left ventricle and indicating LBBB.

Section IV Worksheets

IV.1 HR 83, sinus rhythm. PR interval is 0.16, normal. The QRS is 0.12 seconds indicating BBB. The end of the QRS points to the right in lead I and anteriorly in V1 indicating RBBB. The overall QRS direction is rightward since the S wave in lead I is much bigger than the R wave. This indicates LPHB.

IV.2 Atrial Fibrillation. Ventricular rate is 160. The PR is undefined in a fib. The QRS interval is 0.12 seconds. There is BBB. The end of the QRS is leftward (positive in lead I) and posterior (negative in lead V1) indicating LBBB. Atrial fibrillation may be associated with underlying disease such as cardiomyopathy or heart failure. LBBB is associated with hypertension, coronary disease, and cardiomyopathy.

IV.3 HR 68, sinus. The PR interval is 0.18, normal. The QRS is 0.14 seconds indicating BBB. The end of the QRS is negative in lead I (rightward) and positive in lead V1 (anterior) consistent with

RBBB. The overall QRS points to the patients right, consistent with LPHB. The cause of RBBB and LPHB in this EKG is a septal infarction (Q waves V1 and V2) which is covered in Chapter 15.

IV.4 HR 72. Probable sinus rhythm with PACs and nonconducted PACs. There is not enough information on this EKG to be sure. More rhythm strips are necessary to clarify the rhythm. There is first degree AV block. The QRS interval is greater than 0.12 seconds, so BBB is present. The end of the QRS is positive in lead I and negative in V1 indicating LBBB. Clinically the rhythm needs to be proven, and the cause of LBBB determined.

IV.5 Atrial fibrillation. Ventricular rate 80. QRS interval is 0.11 indicating IVCD. The end of the QRS is slightly negative in lead I, and positive in lead V1. This is RIVCD (or incomplete RBBB). The overall QRS is pointing upward indicating left anterior hemiblock (LAHB).

Section V

Chapter 13

13.1 HR 79, sinus rhythm. The PR is 0.16 to 0.18. The QRS is 0.08, normal. The QT is 0.40. QTc is 0.460 which is high. The T waves are abnormal and point away from the septum (V1 and V2), and anterior (V3) walls. Since this is the only EKG, the First Rule of the T Wave applies. There is ischemic heart disease, but it may be ischemia or infarction, and new or old. Said another way, clinically there may be an old NSTEMI, a new NSTEMI, or unstable angina. More information is needed.

13.2 HR 77. Rhythm sinus. PR is normal. QRS is 0.10 and ends rightward indicating RIVCD. The P direction is normal. The overall QRS direction is normal. The T direction is abnormal, and points away from the inferior wall since it is negative or inverted in leads II, III, and AVF. Since this is the only EKG available, the first rule of the T wave applies. This may represent an old MI, a new MI, or unstable angina.

13.3 HR 65, sinus rhythm. PR is normal. The QRS interval is normal. The P and QRS directions are normal. The T direction is abnormal and points away from the septum (V1 and V2) and anterior (V3 and V4) consistent with ischemia or infarction. This may represent an old or new event. (First Rule of the T Waves) Less commonly, inverted T waves in leads V1–V3 can be pointing away from the free wall of the right ventricle as might occur in pulmonary hypertension and acute pulmonary embolism.

Chapter 14

14.1 HR 88, sinus. PR interval is normal. QRS interval is difficult to measure but may be 0.12 seconds or more indicating BBB. Since the end of the QRS points anteriorly in V1 it would be RBBB. There is ST elevation in leads V2 through V6 consistent with STEMI. The likely diagnosis is an occlusive thrombus in the LAD. The overall QRS direction is upward indicating LAHB. Both RBBB and LAHB can be complications of acute anterior wall MI, since both the right and left bundle are in the septum. Therapy is aimed at emergent opening of the artery by angioplasty or thrombolysis.

14.2 HR 115, sinus tachycardia. This may represent shock or CHF. The PR interval is normal. The QRS is normal at 0.08 seconds. The QT is 0.320 seconds. The QTc is 0.44 which is high. There is ST elevation in leads V1–V4. By the Third Rule of the T Waves, ST elevation in two contiguous leads takes precedence over the ST depression in II, III, and AVF, which represents reciprocal changes. Therapy is aimed at immediate opening of the artery by angioplasty or thrombolysis.

14.3 The HR is 75, sinus rhythm. The PR interval is long, 0.28, indicating 1°AVB, which is a complication of inferior wall MI. There is ST elevation in II, III, and AVF indicating STEMI. The Third Rule of the T Wave applies, and the ST elevation takes precedence over the ST depression in leads I and AVL. Therapy is aimed at immediate opening of the artery supplying the inferior wall, typically the RCA.

Chapter 15

15.1 HR 100. Sinus Rhythm. PR 0.12, normal. QRS 0.08, normal. QT and QTc normal. P direction normal. QRS upward, but not enough for LAHB. T and ST segments are normal. The initial QRS is abnormal in V1 through V4, consistent with Q wave infarction. Since the ST and T segments are normal, the Q wave infarction may be old. The HR of 100 suggests the possibility of CHF secondary to LV systolic dysfunction after the MI.

15.2 HR 79, sinus rhythm. PR 0.12 seconds. QRS 0.09. QT 0.36. P direction normal. QRS direction normal. Significant Q waves in leads II, III and AVF. This indicates Q wave infarction of the inferior wall. The tall wide R wave in lead V2 is equivalent to a posterior wall Q wave. As to timing, the ST segment depression means the Q wave infarction may have been recent. If this is the only EKG, the First Rule of the T Waves still applies, and the ST depression may be due to the old Q wave infarction, or a new episode of ischemia or infarction. More information is necessary.

15.3 HR 94. Sinus rhythm. Significant Q waves are present in leads V1 through V4. The presence of ST elevation in V1 through V3 takes precedence over everything else (STEMI) and suggests the acuteness of the infarction.

Section V Worksheets

V.1 HR 60 Sinus rhythm. Normal PR and QRS intervals. Normal QT and QTc. Normal P and overall QRS direction. Q waves are present in leads II, III, and AVF. The Q wave in lead II is borderline, but significant in leads III and AVF. There is a wide tall R wave in lead V2 equivalent to a posterior Q wave. This indicates an inferior posterior infarction. The ST segments are normal, so the infarction may be old.

V.2 HR 83. Rhythm sinus. PR and QRS intervals are normal. QT and QTc are normal. ST elevation in leads V2 through V5 takes precedence over everything else. It indicates STEMI. The Q waves indicate infarction and some permanent loss of LV has already occurred.

V.3 HR 103, sinus tachycardia. PR 0.18 normal. The QRS is 0.12 indicating BBB. The end of the QRS is right and anterior indicating RBBB. The overall QRS points to the right indicating LPHB. The ST segments are abnormal in V2 through V6 consistent with ischemia or infarction. The ST segments in RBBB point typically away from the end of the QRS. In this example, the ST segments are not secondary to RBBB, but suggest ischemia or infarction (Rule I). The ST segments should always be checked in RBBB.

V.4 HR 81. Sinus rhythm. Significant Q waves are present in II, III, and AVF. The tall wide R wave in lead V2 is equivalent to a posterior Q wave. The ST segments suggest the timing of the Q waves is recent. If this is the only EKG, the First Rule of the T Waves still raises the possibility that the ST segment changes are new, representing new infarction, or angina.

V.5 HR 75, Sinus Rhythm. PR normal. QRS normal. ST Elevation in II, III, and AVF. The ST depression in leads V2 through V4 may represent a posterior ST elevation equivalent. Regardless, Rule Three of the T Waves applies. Since ST elevation is present in two contiguous leads, it takes precedence over the ST segment depression. Therapy should be directed immediately to opening the closed artery.

Section VI

Chapter 16

16.1 HR 115 sinus tachycardia. PR interval is 0.12 seconds. The QRS is 0.08, normal. The QT measures 0.32. The QTc is 0.44 which is high. The P direction is normal. The QRS direction is upward, indicating LAHB. There are tall P waves in leads II, III, and AVF indicating right atrial abnormality. There is a borderline left atrial abnormality as well. There is poor R wave progression in leads V1 to V3. This may represent infarction or may possibly be due to COPD.

16.2 Sinus tachycardia, rate 107. Normal PR and QRS intervals. Normal P direction. QRS direction is leftward but not inferior, which is nonspecific. There are tall P waves in leads II, III, and AVF indicating right atrial abnormality. There is ST segment depression in leads V2 through V4. If only this EKG is available the ST segment changes may represent ischemia or infarction, and may be new or old. More information is necessary (Rule I of T waves).

16.3 HR 71. Rhythm sinus. PR interval is 0.20 seconds. QRS interval is 0.09 seconds. The QT is 0.40. The QTc is normal. The P direction and QRS direction are normal. There are diffuse ST segment changes. (Check the ST in III and V6 with a straight edge.) On a single EKG they may represent ischemia or infarction, and be new or old. There are criteria for both right and left atrial abnormalities.

Chapter 17

17.1 Sinus bradycardia. PAC's are present which are nonconducted, leading to pauses. There are voltage criteria for LVH. There is ST segment depression. This may be due to LVH, ischemia, or infarction. The most likely cause of LVH is hypertension, which is also a primary risk factor for the development of coronary artery disease. The presence of LVH would indicate the development of hypertensive heart disease. Other causes of LVH are pressure and volume overload states on the left ventricle. Although the ST segments may be secondary to LVH, they may also represent ischemia or infarction (Rule I of T waves). More information is necessary.

17.2 HR 88. Sinus rhythm. Right atrial abnormality. Left atrial abnormality. LVH. ST changes consistent with LVH or ischemia or infarction.

17.3 HR 60. Sinus rhythm. LVH. Diffuse nonspecific ST changes consistent with LVH or ischemia or infarction. (Check the ST in III and V6 with a straight edge.)

Chapter 18

18.1 HR 150, sinus tachycardia with a PAC. The QRS is rightward indicating RVH, or LPHB. There is an SI QTIII pattern suggestive of pulmonary embolism. There is diffuse ST segment depression (Rule I of the T waves applies).

18.2 HR 75, sinus rhythm. QT 0.40. QTc is high. The QRS direction is anterior (positive in V1 and V2) indicating RVH.

18.3 HR 115, sinus tachycardia. Right and left atrial abnormality are present. The QRS direction is rightward indicating RVH, or LPHB. The combination of LAA, RAA, and RVH suggests mitral stenosis, with right sided hypertrophy.

Section VI Worksheets

VI.1 HR 75, sinus. PR normal. QRS 0.09, normal. Normal P and QRS direction. Q waves in leads V1 through V4 consistent with Q wave infarction, possibly old. There is a left atrial abnormality. The QRS voltage is high possibly representing LVH. There are nonspecific ST changes diffusely. (Check with straight edge.)

VI.2 Sinus arrhythmia. Left atrial abnormality. LVH. Diffuse ST segment changes consistent with LVH or ischemia or infarction. ST elevation in V3 and V4 takes precedence (Third Rule).

VI.3 Sinus rhythm at 71. SI Q III pattern suggests possibility of pulmonary embolism. Anterior T wave changes consistent with septal ischemia or infarction (Rule One of the T Waves), or acute pulmonary hypertension. The high QRS voltage in V3 and V4 may represent LVH as well.

VI.4 Sinus tachycardia. HR 107. The QRS direction is rightward in lead I indicating RVH, or LPHB. The QRS direction is anterior in V1 also indicating RVH. There are also voltage criteria for LVH. Leads V3 and V4 have tall R and S waves, which also suggest biventricular hypertrophy.

VI.5 HR 88. Baseline artifact is present but the rhythm is sinus. The PR interval is long, 1° AV Block. LVH with ST changes consistent with LVH ischemia or infarction.

Section VII

Chapter 19

19.1 Atrial fibrillation. Low voltage. Low amplitude T waves. QT 0.44 QTc high. Diffuse nonspecific ST changes. Suggestive of hypokalemia. Serum potassium was 2.3 mEq/liter.

19.2 HR 65. QT 0.50. The QTc is 0.52 and dangerously long. Diffuse ST segment changes, possibly secondary to drug or electrolyte effects. Hypokalemia and hypocalcemia should be ruled out immediately. The cause, drug or electrolyte should be identified and corrected.

19.3 Hyperkalemia. Sine wave pattern. Diagnostic and requires immediate therapy to lower the serum potassium level.

Chapter 20

20.1 Diffuse wide QRS in sine wave pattern. Hyperkalemia.

20.2 Sinus Tachycardia. RVH. SI QT III pattern. Rule out pulmonary embolism. Diffuse ST segment depression, so Rule I of the T waves also applies.

20.3 LBBB

Section VII Worksheets

VII.1 HR 100, sinus rhythm. QT 0.44. The QTc is 0.57 which is dangerously long. Drug and electrolyte abnormalities must be identified immediately and corrected. Diffuse ST changes present (Rule I also applies).

VII.2 Sinus tachycardia. RVH. Inferior Q waves. SI QT III pattern. Acute pulmonary embolism should be ruled out. Peaked T waves, rule out hyperkalemia.

VII.3 Low voltage. There is dramatic reduction of voltage. Pneumothorax, COPD, pericardial effusion, pleural effusion, should be considered. This patient had infiltrative cardiomyopathy.

VII.4 Peaked T waves in V2 and V3. Hyperkalemia.

VII.5 LBBB with a very wide QRS. This combination suggests additional conduction depression from drug or electrolyte effect.

Section VIII

Self-Assessment Worksheets

VIII.1 Sinus rhythm. Rate 71. PR 0.18. QRS 0.10, IVCD. Right atrial abnormality. Left atrial abnormality. LVH. Pressure or volume overload of the LV, most commonly due to hypertension. Diffuse ST changes due to LVH or ischemia or infarction.

VIII.2 1°AV Block, LBBB. Associations include coronary disease, hypertension, and cardiomyopathy.

VIII.3 RBBB. LPHB. ST changes are expected for RBBB.

VIII.4 Peaked T waves indicate hyperkalemia. (K^+ was 7.8)

VIII.5 Sine wave of hyperkalemia. (K^+ was 8.5)

VIII.6 Sinus rhythm with PAC and ST elevation in the inferior, anterior, and lateral walls. Rule Three of the T Waves. The ST elevation takes precedence over the ST segment depression (which represents reciprocal changes). Immediate evaluation for possible angioplasty or thrombolysis is appropriate. (STEMI)

VIII.7 SI Q T III pattern of pulmonary embolism.

VIII.8 Atrial fibrillation. SI Q T III pattern. Anterior ST depression indicates septal or right ventricular free wall ischemia.

VIII.9 Inferior Q waves indicate inferior Q wave infarction, possibly recently since the ST segments are abnormal. Wide R wave in V2 indicates posterior MI or RVH.

VIII.10 Delta wave and short PR interval indicate WPW.